THE HEALTH OF NATIONS

Also by the authors

THE SOCIETY AND POPULATION
HEALTH READER, VOL. I
(EDITED BY THE AUTHORS
AND RICHARD G. WILKINSON)

THE HEALTH OF NATIONS

Why Inequality Is Harmful to Your Health

ICHIRO KAWACHI AND BRUCE P. KENNEDY

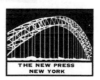

THE NEW PRESS
NEW YORK

Published in the United States by The New Press, New York, 2002
Distributed by W. W. Norton & Company, Inc., New York

LIBRARY OF CONGRESS CATALOGING-IN-PUBLICATION DATA
Kawachi, Ichiro.
The health of nations : why inequality is harmful to your health/
Ichiro Kawachi and Bruce P. Kennedy.
p.   cm.
Includes bibliographical references and index.
ISBN 1-56584-582-X (hc.)
1. Medical care—Social aspects.   2. Medical policy—Social aspects.
3. Health services accessibility.   4. Social medicine.
5. Equality—Health aspects.   I. Kennedy, Bruce P.   II. Title.

RA418.5.P6 K39 2002

362.1—dc21   2001056276

The New Press was established in 1990 as a not-for-profit alternative to the large,
commercial publishing houses currently dominating the book publishing industry.
The New Press operates in the public interest rather than for private gain,
and is committed to publishing, in innovative ways, works of educational,
cultural, and community value that are often deemed insufficiently profitable.

The New Press, 450 West 41st Street, 6th floor, New York, NY 10036
www.thenewpress.com

Book design by Lovedog Studio

Composition by dix!

Printed in the United States of America

2   4   6   8   10   9   7   5   3   1

CONTENTS

ACKNOWLEDGMENTS

We owe an intellectual debt to our colleague Richard Wilkinson, whose pioneering ideas on the social consequences of inequality shaped our own thinking on the subject. This book is the end product of numerous conversations and debates we have had with him over the past five years. Alvin Tarlov and Barbara Kimivae Krimgold, who together ran the Robert Wood Johnson Investigator Awards in Health Policy Research, were instrumental in putting us in touch with our publisher, André Schiffrin, of The New Press. We only wish we had just half the level of energy and enthusiasm with which Barbara has championed the cause of reducing disparities. If this book succeeds in moving the debate a little further into the public realm, it is because of the tireless prodding and encouragement of Al and Andre.

During the course of writing this book, we have also benefited immeasurably from the exchange of ideas with colleagues. We would especially like to thank our colleagues in the Mac-

Arthur Foundation Network on Socioeconomic Status and Health (Nancy Adler, Michael Marmot, Katherine Newman, Bruce McEwen, David Williams, Sheldon Cohen, Karen Matthews, Teresa Seeman, Shelley Taylor, Mark Cullen, and Joel Schwartz), and the Harvard Center for Society and Health (Lisa Berkman, Kimberly Lochner, S. V. Subramanian, Tony Blakely, Laura Kubzansky, Nancy Krieger, and Jody Heymann).

It has been a special privilege to meet and exchange ideas with our colleagues around the world. Daniel Reidpath of Deakin University (Melbourne, Australia) found the advertising data in Chapter 4. Philippa Howden Chapman of the Wellington School of Medicine, New Zealand, supplied the pithy quote from Seneca in the Introduction. My students in the short course on social epidemiology in Australia drew my attention to the baseball data in Chapter 5. We thank Tony Casas and Norberto Dachs, of the Pan American Health Organization, for pushing us to think about the global dimensions of inequality. Our colleagues in the Robert Wood Johnson Investigator Awards program have been wonderful sounding boards for our ideas—we especially thank the political scientists (Larry Jacobs, Jim Morone, and Mark Peterson), and also Norman Daniels, Jim House, Bruce Link and Jo Phelan, Deborah and Rodrick Wallace, and Dick Levins. Bob Putnam, whose ideas on social capital and civic engagement appear throughout this book, has been a constant source of inspiration. Last but not least, this book represents the latest (but by no means the last) product of a journey that Sol Levine, our mentor, sent us off on. Though he passed away prematurely in 1996, his spirit of inquiry lives on.

Ichiro would like to thank his wife, Cathy. Chunks of this book were written during the happy sleepless nights following the birth of their daughter Kate.

—*Ichiro Kawachi and Bruce Kennedy*
Boston, November 2000

INTRODUCTION

Occurrent, quod genus egestatis gravissimum est, in divitiis inopes.

"You will know of those who are poor in the midst of riches, which is the worst of poverties."
—SENECA, *Epistles to Lucilius,* 88.28

We live in a vastly unequal world. Over a billion people around the world eke out a living on incomes of $1 a day, or less. Three-fifths of the world's people in the poorest sixty-one countries receive just 6 percent of the world's income—or less than $2 a day per person. Meanwhile, in the U.S.A., the wealthiest country in the world, automobiles and houses are getting bigger. Buoyed by the most recent economic boom, the net worth of the median American household rose to $71,600 in 1998, up 17.6 percent from 1995 (*The New York Times,* January 19, 2000). Near the top of the economic pyramid, the number of millionaires in this country ballooned to one in twenty-five households. Between 1995 and 1998, about 1 million new millionaires were minted, compared with the previous seven-year period during which the number of households with such wealth stayed relatively constant at just over 3 million.

Just how unequal is the world? As midnight approached on the last day of the millennium, a billion television viewers worldwide caught a glimpse of the stark differences in living standards across the globe. On the island republic of Kiribati (gross domestic product, $425 per capita), where the first countdown to the new millennium took place, camera crews descended on a dark beach, where a few dozen revelers chanted songs and swayed in grass skirts. The native dancers appeared oblivious for the moment to a United Nations report that predicted a decade ago that the thirty-three-island nation would eventually disappear under the sea because of global warming.

Four hours later, President Jiang Zemin of China (GDP, $860 per capita) heralded the new millennium with a speech about his country's glorious future. As if on cue, dozens of shopping centers and department stores across Beijing announced that they would stay open until two A.M. in honor of the momentous occasion. So, in a country where celebrations organized by fancy hotels and restaurants remained out of reach for most average families, crowds thronged the shopping malls to compare the prices of electronic gadgets and wait in line at the cash register.

Another quarter-turn of the earth later, midnight approached the village of Ekambu in Namibia. Too remote for television cameras, we nonetheless have this report filed by an intrepid *New York Times* correspondent:

"As the modern world celebrated the coming of 2000 with confetti and champagne, the Himba people started and ended their day much as they have for nearly 300 years, whistling to their goats, milking their cows and sleeping with the sun. . . . In this village of mud huts, there are no calendars, no electricity, no words in the native language for millennium, computer or Y2K. The nearest telephone is a three-hour drive away" (Swarns, 2000).

Yet the same report also hinted at changes to come, for the Namibian government had recently announced a $550 million dam project that, according to an official from the Ministry of Mines and Energy, promised to "change the whole face of the region. . . . The present culture of the Himba people will gradually disappear. [The Himba] will get cars, get jobs, and go to school like everyone else." As if echoing the sentiments of the government official, a village youth—interviewed in his Adidas jacket and faded Puma sneakers—expresses his hope to the reporter that in 2000, he will get a job, buy a car, and help his family.

Finally, midnight approached New York City, where hundreds of thousands of revelers thronged Times Square, eagerly awaiting the 83,000-watt Waterford crystal ball to drop. They were entertained by more than a thousand musicians, dancers, actors, and puppeteers, and meanwhile restrained by the $65,000 worth of metal barricades brought in by the police for the occasion. Across town, some 1,700 party-goers flocked to the black-tie fund-raiser at the American Museum of Natural History, where more than thirty-five chefs and forty bartenders toiled under the shadow of Hayden Planetarium's brand-new $4 million digital dome. The guests each paid between $500 and $5,000 to sit at the banquet table.

This brief snapshot of the globe merely hints at the extent of inequality in present-day terms. Over history, the gap in living standards between the rich and poor countries has been steadily pulling apart. According to data gathered by the United Nations Development Program (UNDP), the richest country in the

world back in 1820 was Great Britain, with a GDP per capita of
$1,750 in 1990 dollars. Back then, the poorest country in the
world was China (GDP per capita, $523), which Britain hap-
pened to be exploiting at that time. As we know, empires tend to
come and go, and every schoolchild can see from the bar chart
why the twentieth century came to be called the American century.

The value of stock markets in the developed world grew 37
percent in 1999, far outpacing the 3 percent average growth of
the same countries. The combined wealth of investors around

TRENDS IN GLOBAL INEQUALITY
1820–1997

GDP Per Capita (1990 PPP U.S. $000)

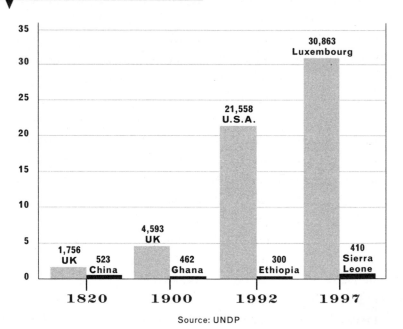

Source: UNDP

the world was $25.5 trillion, with 19 percent growth in Europe and 17 percent in the United States in 1999 alone (Viscusi, 2000).

Just as remarkable as the spectacular rise in living standards of the wealthiest countries has been the stagnation of countries near the bottom. The poorest country in 1997, Sierra Leone, had a *lower* level of GDP in real terms ($410 per capita) than the poorest country back in 1820. Put another way, the income ratio between the richest and poorest countries increased from a three-fold difference in 1820, to over seventy-five-fold a century and a half later. According to the UNDP, economic decline or stagnation has affected nearly one hundred countries in the world since the 1980s, reducing the incomes of 1.6 billion people. In seventy of these countries, average incomes are less than they were in 1980, and in forty-three countries, less than they were in 1970. The average African household consumes 20 percent *less* today than it did twenty-five years ago. About one-third of the children in the world are undernourished.

Inequalities have been growing not just between countries of the world but within individual countries as well. Within the United States, the incomes of the bottom 60 percent of households have stagnated in real terms during the past twenty-five years, whereas the rich have continued to pull ahead. In the mid-1960s, when the economy was growing at about 6 percent per year, the ratio between the income of the top chief executive officers of American corporations and the wage of the average production worker was 39 to 1. In 1997, despite three decades of slower growth, the CEO-worker ratio was 254 to 1 (Faux and Mishel, 2000). The number of U.S. households that earn more than $100,000 a year or have a net worth of more than $500,000—excluding the value of their homes—grew to 16.7

million in 1998, up from 11.7 million in 1996. That is five times the growth of the overall population. The number of "super-rich," those worth more than $5 million, has grown 46 percent *each year* in the past five years (Viscusi, 2000). Last year, it took 100 million of the lowest earning Americans to equal the after-tax dollars of the top *1* percent. Back in 1977, it only took 49 million of the lowest earners to equal the top 1 percent, (*The New York Times,* September 3, 2000, p. WK3). Working families with children are working harder and harder to maintain a decent standard of living. The number of earners per family has increased, as have the number of weeks worked per year, and the number of hours worked per week (Herbert, 2000).

Down at the bottom of the economic heap, we have hardly made a dent on the national poverty rate. Despite the extraordinary economic boom of the 1990s, the number of citizens eking out an existence below the federal poverty level remains at 12.7 percent, just one-tenth of a percentage less than in 1989, and one full percentage higher than in 1979 (Herbert, 2000). One in the five children live in poverty, while 2 million Americans languish in prisons.

So what? Do these inequalities matter in any important sense? Other than causing envy, are there any undesirable consequences of widening disparities in income, wealth, and living standards? Or is inequality the engine for growth, ensuring that the benefits trickle down to those at the bottom? For that matter, why do we care about economic growth? In other words, what is the purpose of economic development? These are the questions we will tackle in this book.

Far from being a benign by-product of capitalism's success, we shall argue that growing inequalities threaten the various freedoms that economic development is supposed to bring about: freedom from want, freedom from ill health, freedom to exercise democratic choice, as well as freedom to pursue leisure and the activities that we have reason to value. This book is not about why some countries enjoy high rates of economic growth while others do not. We leave that subject to economists. What this book is about is why we care about economic development, and how we should evaluate what the economy delivers. The Nobel laureate Amartya Sen has written eloquently on these issues in the context of developing countries. By contrast, the principal focus of our book is on the United States of America. Following the collapse of the centrally planned economies, our government has led the way in foisting our free-market models on the rest of the world. It is timely, then, to take stock and ask: How are we doing?

Economic Goals and "The Permanent Problem of the Human Race"

Living in the Material World

Nineteen ninety-four marked the United Nations' International Year of the Family. To commemorate this occasion, the award-winning photographer Peter Menzel embarked on an ambitious project—to capture the range and diversity of living standards across countries of the world. The quest took the photographer and his team to thirty different countries across four continents, ranging from the extremely poor to the very rich. They visited some of the most destitute nations on the planet: Ethiopia, Bhutan, and Mali, ranked respectively, 180th, 174th, and 162nd out of 183 UN nations in terms of affluence. The team also dropped in on some of the most affluent countries, like the U.S.A., Japan, and Iceland. The resulting book—part photojournalism, part anthropology—depicts ordinary families in poor and rich countries going about their daily business, at work, or interacting with their neighbors and loved ones. At each location, the photographer made one unusual request of his subjects, which was to get them to pose in front of their homes along with all of their material possessions. This meant that for each family portrait, Menzel's subjects literally agreed to haul all their worldly belongings out into the street and display them in front of their house. The result is a pictorial record of all the household furnishings, kitchen utensils, electronic gadgets, toys, and tools that families around the world happened to own at that moment. Menzel's book, aptly titled *Material World: A Global Family Portrait* (Sierra Club Books, 1994), provides an unforgettable visual record of the way people live, but it is also a startling documentary of the contrasts in living standards across the globe. Take three snapshots from three different countries at dramatically different stages of economic development:

From Ethiopia (per capita income $123 per year), we have a portrait of the Getu family—Mr. Getu, his wife, and five children—smiling and seated beneath the blue sky in front of their 320-square-foot thatched-roof, earthen-floor dwelling. Arranged around the family on the dry, chaff-strewn ground are a wooden mortar and pestle (for pounding grain), pots and pans, a bed with a woolen blanket, and an umbrella. These constitute their entire inventory of worldly possessions. The family also keeps two oxen, three horses, a sheep, a goat, and eight chickens, some of which take pride of place alongside family members in the group portrait.

Contrast this with Mexico, a country of intermediate economic development (per capita income $2,971, and ranked 51st in affluence out of 183 UN nations), where the Castillo family lives. The family—father and mother, and their four children—were photographed on the rooftop of their 700-square-foot, two-bedroom cinder-block apartment building in Guadalajara. You can see their washing hanging on the line behind them, catching the last rays of sun on a late August afternoon. The family is seated next to their rooftop vegetable garden, where a few stalks of corn are growing. Behind the Castillos' smiling heads we can see the family possessions spread out in a cramped space between neighboring apartments: a kitchen stove, refrigerator, washing machine, hi-fi stereo, three bicycles, color TV, and a variety of household furnishings.

Moving to the pinnacle of economic development, we arrive at the United States (per capita income $22,356), where the Skeen family—husband and wife, with their two children—stand proudly in front of their 1,600-square-foot ranch house, located in a cul-de-sac in a suburb of Houston, Texas. Spread out across their manicured lawn and spacious driveway are (what must seem to a citizen of the Third World) a bewildering panoply of consumer products. These include three motor vehicles (a Ford F350 pickup, a Ford Aerostar, and a dune buggy), two television sets, three stereo sets, five telephones, a VCR, computer, piano, microwave, dishwasher, washing machine and dryer, and an assortment of furniture and toys (Figure 1.1).

At each of the three locations, the families were also photographed going about their daily chores. In turn, the range of daily activities pursued by each family in different countries closely mirrors the increasing degrees of freedom that material affluence brings. In Ethiopia, every morning, Mr. Getu's wife, Zenebu Tulu, and her eight-year-old daughter, Like, leave their hut to harvest fresh dung from the backyard corral and mix it with straw into paste, some of which is used to plaster the walls of the house. They flatten the rest into patties that are then used for fuel. When fuel is scarce, the whole family scavenges the

FIGURE 1.1

COMPARISON OF LIVING STANDARDS
IN THREE COUNTRIES

Country	Family	Dwelling	Material possessions	Family budget
ETHIOPIA	Mr. Getu (30), Mrs. Getu (25), 5 children (10, 8, 8, 7, 3)	320 sq. ft. thatched-roof, earthen-floor hut	Mortar and pestle, pots and pans, bed and blanket, 2 oxen, 3 horses, sheep, goat, 8 chickens, umbrella	One-third spent on school supplies
MEXICO	Mr. Castillo (29), Mrs. Castillo (25), 4 children (10, 8, 7, 5)	700 sq. ft. 2-bedroom cinder-block apartment	Refrigerator, washing machine, stove, 2 stereos, color TV, 3 beds, 2 couches, 2 tables, dresser, cabinet, wardrobe, arc welder, 3 bicycles, bookcase, kitchen utensils, electric fan, 6 pairs shoes	57 percent spent on food, 28 percent on clothing
U.S.A.	Mr. Skeen (36), Mrs. Skeen (34), 2 children (10, 7)	1,600 sq. ft. ranch house with lawn and 2-car garage	3 cars (truck, van, dune buggy), 2 TV's, VCR, 3 stereos, 1 computer, 5 telephones, washer-dryer, refrigerator, dishwasher, range, microwave, piano, dining table and 6 chairs, 3 beds, couch, 2 dressers, 2 cabinets, desk, 2 sewing machines, 4 bicycles, rifle, shotgun, trampoline (*partial list*)	9 percent spent on food

Source: Menzel

nearby fields. We see a picture of little Like, returning from a day in the fields, precariously balancing on top of her head a platter piled high with cow dung. Working with dung takes up much of the daily work-hours of the women in the Getu household. The Getus live only two hours by car from Addis Ababa, Ethiopia's modern capital, yet in their village they have no running water, no plumbing, no electricity. The only hint of urbanization, according to the notes jotted down by the photographer, consists of the high-tension wires that run through the valley behind the Getus' dwelling, on their way from a hydroelectric project to the capital. Local schooling is free, but the children are required to buy their own clothes and supplies that would consume perhaps a third of the family's annual budget. All told, fewer than a hundred children attend the school in the Getus' village, in a catchment area of more than ten thousand people. Asked what their wishes are for the future, the Getus reply "more animals, a second set of clothes, better seed stock, farm implements, and peace in the area and in the world."

In Guadalajara, Mexico, the walled courtyard behind the Castillo household is the focus of the family's daily activities. It is where Mr. Castillo keeps his welding equipment for his free-lance welding jobs (he also works a day job at a wholesale produce distributor, where he loads crates of produce for sixteen hours a day, starting at 4:00 A.M.). The courtyard is also where his wife keeps the washing machine, which is connected to the public water main by a garden hose. Though the interior of the Castillo home bears the familiar markings of twentieth-century comfort (an upholstered sofa, linoleum floors, and an electric fan), just beyond the parents' upstairs bedroom, the doorway opens onto a ten-foot drop, where Mr. Castillo has not had the time to construct the requisite stairs. For now, the family climbs up through a hole in the floor on a cramped temporary spiral staircase welded together by Mr. Castillo. During the time that the photographer stayed with the family, they take a trip on the bus to downtown Guadalajara for a shopping expedition. The children, especially the two girls, are dressed in their Sunday best: floral pattern dresses with pink sashes and lace sleeves. The parents indulge them with new shoes, school backpacks, and ice-cream cones for all. The family spends 57 percent of their annual income on food, and another 28 percent on clothing. Asked what their wishes are for the future, they answer "a truck."

Meantime, in the suburb of Houston, where the Skeens live, it is approaching Thanksgiving, and Mrs. Skeen is photographed at the local supermarket, where she is stocking up for the big meal. Behind her shopping cart we catch a familiar glimpse of supermarket shelves filled to bursting with different cuts of meat—ground beef, blade steak, tenderloin, Porter-house, rib-eye, T-bone—as well as the neatly arranged stacks of prepackaged, presliced, processed cheeses. The Skeens spend just 9 percent of their family budget on food. Mr. Skeen works as a cable splicer, and Mrs. Skeen works half-time as a teacher at a Christian academy. After a hard day at work, Mr. and Mrs. Skeen are photographed relaxing in their living room in front of their twenty-inch color television set, where a Dallas Cowboys game is in progress. Mr. Skeen owns several rifles, and his hobby is to hunt for deer, not for the meat but for the trophies. His living room is decorated with a stuffed deer's head and two sets of antlers (beside a wall of family portraits). Asked what their wishes are for the future, they reply, "tools, new carpet, camper trailer."

The message of Menzel's book is as simple as it is stark. In spite of reaching the moon, achieving the global eradication of polio, supplying the remotest corners of the earth with electricity and the Internet, drastic inequalities in living standards persist (indeed, continue to widen) across the planet. Based on the visual evidence presented by Peter Menzel's survey, there can be no gainsaying that more purchasing power could improve the quality of life of poor people on the planet.

But how much more, and how do we judge what is sufficient? Should the consumption standards of a country like the United States be held up to the rest of the world as an example for other countries to emulate?

UNBALANCED CONSUMPTION: THE CASE OF WORLD HUNGER

The historian David Landes has remarked that the world can be divided roughly into three kinds of nations: those that spend lots of money to keep their weight down; those whose people eat to live; and those whose people don't know where the next meal is coming from (Landes, 1998). The United States is one of those nations that spends lots of money to keep its waistlines down. The diet-advice industry—a market of books, programs, foods, and other weight-related products—nets over $34 billion each year, not to mention the sums Americans spend on surgery to trim excess fat (Vogel, 1999). Some 32 million American women and 26 million men—about one-third of the adult population—are overweight as a result of excessive caloric intake and sedentary lifestyles encouraged by television-watching, automobile transportation, and remote-control buttons on entertainment gadgets. The extra health-care costs of treating the morbidity attributed to obesity (diabetes, hypertension, heart disease, arthritis) amounted to $51.6 billion in 1995, or about 5.7 percent of our nation's total health-care expenditure (Wolf and Colditz, 1998). Contrast this pattern of nutritional excess with the estimate that about 1 billion of the world's 5 billion people are chronically hungry, with many dying from lack of food or suffering from diseases born of malnutrition (Bradshaw and Wallace, 1996). Upward of forty thousand children die each day from hunger-related causes (Kloby, 1997).

The problem is not that there isn't enough food to feed everyone on the planet. The world produces enough grain to provide everyone with 3,600 calories per day. The problem is that the world's food consumption patterns are wildly out of balance. The richest countries of the world where a quarter of the earth's population live—including the United States, Canada, Japan, and those of Western Europe—consume 70 percent of the world's food grains. Much of the grains "consumed" by rich countries are actually used to feed beef and dairy cattle. The average American consumes about two thousand pounds of grain per year, most of it in the form of milk, eggs, meat, and alcoholic beverages. Americans each consume an average of 260 pounds of meat per year. On current estimates, it takes about twenty pounds of grain to produce each pound of beef. Contrast this with the average Bangladeshi who consumes just 6.5 pounds of meat per year (Kloby, 1997). A significant amount of the food in the developed world goes to waste. North American families waste 10 to 15 percent of the food they buy (Rathje and Murphy, 1992). Beyond feeding themselves, Americans and Europeans spend $17 billion a year on pet food—$4 billion more than the estimated annual total needed to provide basic health and nutrition for everyone in the world (UNDP, 1998).

The problem of world hunger, therefore, is not due to absolute food shortage, but rather due to inequalities in the *distribution* of food. According to Oxfam, many of the world's poorest nations are net exporters of food. Thirty-six of the world's poorest nations export food to North America. Africa, where more than half of the population suffers from malnutrition, exports millions of dollars' worth of food to Europe each year. Likewise, India is one of the top Third World food exporters, even though 300 million Indians go hungry each day. The world's second largest food exporter is Brazil, where 86 million suffer from hunger (Kloby, 1997).

Because of these inequalities, the eradication of world hunger is unlikely to be accomplished by simply exhorting poor countries to grow more food and pull themselves out of poverty. Part of the blame for persistent hunger and poverty in the Third World must rest with the First World and its excesses. Sadly, on current trends, there seems little hope that the First World is prepared to downshift its consumption habits to more sustainable and equitable levels; whereas there is every indication that the rest of the world is determined to catch up to and imitate the standards set by the west. One of the more unsettling coincidences uncovered by Menzel's research was that, in impoverished communities across the globe, from China to Thailand to Uzbekistan, when families were asked about their wishes for the future, so many replied: "A second television set." Not safe drinking water, not childhood immunizations, but a color television set. Critics of western consumer societies maintain that poor people and poor countries make inappropriate decisions about what to consume, and reduce their savings and investment because they are misled by seeing the consumption patterns of richer people and nations (Goodwin, et al., 1997).

Champions of the free market dismiss such claims on the grounds that when it comes to choices over what and how much to spend, the consumer is sovereign. Yet those of us lucky enough to be born in North America may wonder what kind of a planet we would live in if every Chinese or Indian family aspired to the living standard of Americans, where 62 percent of households drive two or more cars; and 92 percent own at least one vehicle.

Global inequalities have not only persisted but have actually gotten worse over time, thereby raising the stakes for less-developed nations to catch up to the ever-rising standards of living set by the affluent countries. Today, it is estimated that the richest 20 percent of the world account for 86 percent of total private consumption expenditures, while the poorest 20 percent account for a minuscule 1.3 percent (UNDP, 1998).

"THE PERMANENT PROBLEM OF THE HUMAN RACE"

After the last fireworks had gone off on the last day of the twentieth century, after all the confetti had settled, the millions of tired citizens went home to sleep, to make New Year's resolutions (to lose weight?), and to pray for prosperity in the new millennium. Let us pause for a moment to consider this last fact. It is universally accepted by now that human beings throughout the world, no matter what their differences in culture or material circumstances, wish for greater prosperity and higher living standards. But greater prosperity to do what? To acquire more material possessions? Or, more likely, to attain happiness that the acquisition of material goods is supposed to bring?

The yawning gulf in living standards across the globe, and

the seemingly insatiable quest for more material possessions, raise questions about what *ought* to be the goal of economic development. In a famous essay written during the Great Depression, John Maynard Keynes pondered this very question:

> Let us, for the sake of argument, suppose that a hundred years hence we are all of us, on the average, eight times better off in the economic sense than we are to-day. Assuredly there need be nothing here to surprise us.
>
> Now it is true that the needs of human beings may seem to be insatisable. But they fall into two classes—those needs which are absolute in the sense that we feel them whatever the situation of our fellow human beings may be, and those which are relative in the sense that we feel them only if their satisfaction lifts us above, makes us feel superior to, our fellows. Needs of the second class, those which satisfy the desire for superiority, may indeed by insatiable; for the higher the general level, the higher still are they. But this is not so true of the absolute needs—a point may soon be reached, much sooner perhaps than we are all of us aware of, when these needs are satisfied in the sense that we prefer to devote our further energies to non-economic purposes (Keynes, 1931, p. 365)

From this simple thought experiment, Keynes concluded that "the *economic problem* may be solved, or be at least within sight of solution, within a hundred years," which meant that "the economic problem is not—if we look into the future—*the permanent problem of the human race*" (emphasis in the original).

In other words, *what if* the real problem, "the permanent problem of the human race," turns out not be economic growth *per se,* but learning how to use the freedom from pressing economic wants, how to occupy the leisure freed up by economic progress, in short, learning how to "live wisely and agreeably and well"? If by "living well" we mean a better quality of life, then what is the evidence that our economic priorities have in fact delivered the things we really value? And how should we measure the quality of life? By levels of consumption, per capita gross national product, the attainment of happiness, or some other yardstick?

These are the broad questions addressed in this book. Because of America's influential position in the world economy— as producer, consumer, and trading partner—much of the evidence and arguments in this book will focus on the American case. Because fixing the problem of global inequalities requires first that we put our own house in order, we shall pay special attention to the successes and failures of the American way of life. We pose the question whether our recent economic performance deserves to be the envy of the world, and whether our economy is indeed taking us in a direction that the rest of the world would want to follow.

JUDGING THE GREAT AMERICAN GROWTH MACHINE

The American economy may be likened to an engine whose smooth functioning is tracked by indicators such as the Consumer Price Index, the Industrial Production Index, or the Dow Jones Index. Obviously any poor performance calls for repairs; and it is the job of a good mechanic (perhaps Federal Reserve Chairman Alan Greenspan—at least according to the *Wall Street Journal*) to avoid breakdowns and ensure the good condition of the engine. But keeping the engine trouble-free is not an end in itself. The engine drives a vehicle, and it is the direction in which the vehicle is traveling that really matters. Are Americans content with the general direction in which the economy is headed? A variety of evidence suggests otherwise. The welfare of our citizens—whether measured by happiness or good health—has stagnated and steadily departed from the growth trajectory traced by economic indicators like the Dow-Jones average or even GNP per capita. Contrary to claims that "the Great American Growth Machine continues to deliver what we want" (Cox and Alm, 1999), we argue that the direction our economy is taking has not improved the quality of life of our citizens.

Some economists might object that being happy and healthy are not the only goals that Americans value. But when asked what *is* the goal of our economic activities, the economist's stock response is "to maximize utility." Pressed further, however, most economists concede that utility is practically undefinable, and they resort instead to the yardstick of "maximizing consumption" as a proxy (Goodwin, 1997). According to this view, our level of welfare is most accurately reflected by what we consume. The bigger our cars and the more spacious our homes, the higher our standard of living, and ergo, the higher must be our level of social welfare. But is the maximization of consumption what we *really* want? Is consumption a good yardstick for social welfare?

Far from delivering what people want, we argue that our present patterns of consumption are less than optimal, and may actually threaten the long-term well-being of individuals and society, indeed of the globe. Far from being a sign of national progress, the growth of our consumer culture conceals a deep underlying pathology, namely, the widening rift between the haves and have-nots. Growing disparities in income, and the relative deprivation it engenders, has forced American families to leap on the treadmill of overwork, declining leisure, declining community participation, and spending decisions (financed by debt) that contribute less and less to the welfare of individuals, society, and the world at large.

From 1983 to 1995, the gross domestic product of America grew by 41 percent in real terms, or about $1,000 per employee. Has this record of growth made America the envy of the western world? The answer is not at all obvious if we take into account the fact that starting in the mid-1970s, the economic performance of the United States has been blemished by a steadily widening gulf between rich and poor. Until the early 1980s, interest in the distribution of earnings and incomes was regarded as a parochial backwater in economic research (Gottschalk and Smeeding, 1997). This lack of interest reflected the view that the distribution of income in the United States and elsewhere showed little change between the end of the 1940s and the mid-1970s. One economist went so far as to remark in 1978 that tracking changes in the distribution of income in the United States "was like watching the grass grow" (Aaron, 1978). Between 1947 and 1973, American families at every step of the economic ladder enjoyed income growth— and the poorest families had the highest rate of all.

But, beginning in 1973, the economy began registering sharp increases in both earnings and income inequality. Since then, the affluent sections of society have been pulling away sharply from the middle class and poor (Shapiro and Greenstein, 1999). Between 1977 and 1999, the average after-tax incomes of the top fifth of American families rose by 43 percent. By contrast, the average incomes of the middle fifth of families rose by a meager 8 percent over the same twenty-two-year period, or less than 0.5

percent per year. At the bottom, the incomes of poor families actually fell by 9 percent. Forty percent of American families are either no better off or worse off today in real terms than they were back in 1977. But at the very top, the incomes of the wealthiest *1 percent* of the population rose by a whopping 115 percent after adjusting for inflation (Figure 1.2).

FIGURE 1.2

PERCENTAGE CHANGE IN AFTER-TAX INCOME, 1977 TO 1999

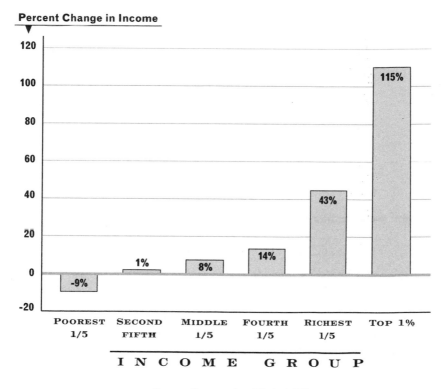

Source: Congressional Budget Office

Income disparities have widened to such a degree that in 1999, the top 1 percent of the population received as much after-tax income as the bottom 38 percent combined. The 2.7 million Americans with the largest incomes thus received as much after-tax income as the bottom 100 million Americans (Shapiro and Greenstein, 1999). In case the reader is wondering how much after-tax income was needed in 1999 to make it to the top 20 percent, the figure was $102,300; and $515,600 to make it into the top 1 percent. The extent of income inequality today is at the widest level on record since the Congressional Budget Office began collecting statistics more than twenty years ago.

Wealth has become concentrated in even fewer hands. (Wealth refers to the net dollar value of the stock of assets minus debts held by a household at one point in time, as distinct from income, which refers to the flow of dollars over a year.) In the early part of this century, inequality in the distribution of wealth was much lower in the United States than in the United Kingdom, and comparable to levels in Sweden. As the economist Edward Wolff (1996) pointed out: "America appeared to be the land of opportunity, whereas Europe was a place where an entrenched upper class controlled the bulk of wealth." By the end of the 1980s, however, America suffered from a far higher concentration of wealth than Europe. It is Europe that now appears like the land of equality. On current estimates, the wealthiest 1 percent of American society owns 48 percent of the nation's financial assets, and 39 percent of the nation's total assets, including real estate (Wolff, 1995; Hacker, 1997). After the stock market crash of 1929, inequality in wealth was on a downward drift that lasted until the late 1970s. But since then, inequality of wealth holdings, like that of income, has risen sharply. Between 1983 and 1989, the share of wealth owned by the top 1 percent increased by 5 percent, while the share held by the bottom 80 percent fell by more than 20 percent. Notwithstanding estimates that some 45 million American families, or 44 percent of American households, now own a share of the stock market, the top 1 percent of households is still estimated to hold nearly half of the stocks by value, while the bottom 90 percent owns just 14 percent (Wolff, 1996).

The four hundred richest Americans, annually anointed by *Forbes* magazine, were collectively worth $1 trillion in 1999, more than the gross domestic product of China (Galewitz, 1999). The minimum net worth needed to qualify for the Forbes 400 list was $625 million in 1999, up from $550 million in 1998. Of the 400 individuals listed, more than half (268) were in fact billionaires. Nearly 40 percent of the names on the list got rich the easy way—i.e., by inheritance. On the other hand, the rest of them made their fortunes through hard work, innovation, and ability—qualities that Americans widely admire and aspire to. So why fuss about widening disparities in income and wealth?

In point of fact, Americans seem to care rather little about income disparity compared with citizens in other parts of the world. The level of income disparities in this country is the highest in the league of economically advanced nations. Figure 1.3 displays the extent of income disparities in twenty-two economically advanced countries, taken from the Luxembourg Income Study (Smeeding, 1998). The measure of income inequality is the so-called decile ratio, which is the ratio of the income of a person in the top 10 percent of the population compared with the level of income of a person in the bottom 10 percent (where income levels have been indexed to the median income in each country). The greater the length of the bar on Figure 1.3, the greater the social distance between the top

and bottom of the economic hierarchy. As can be seen, the
United States is an extreme case.

When citizens of different countries have been polled about
attitudes toward income inequality, Americans come out near
the bottom in their dislike of wide disparities. According to a
World Values survey conducted in the early nineties, only 38
percent of Americans responded favorably to a question about
the desirability of policies to reduce income inequalities, compared with 65 percent in Great Britain (the lowest among European countries), and nearly 80 percent in Italy (the most
egalitarian respondents) (Lipset, 1997). Proportionately fewer
Americans (56 percent) agree that "income differences are too
large," as compared with Europeans (whose responses ranged
from 66 to 86 percent). Strikingly, even the poor in America are
less likely to endorse redistributive or egalitarian sentiments
than low-income citizens elsewhere.

To be sure, our country has been racked by occasional fits of
concern about the income gulf, especially during periods of
economic downturns. But on the whole, we seem curiously content to watch these inequalities grow. In point of fact, virtually
every economic policy initiative introduced during recent years
seems to be designed to widen these inequalities still further. As
a nation, we seem to be hooked on policy proposals to balance
the budget, trim the income tax, roll back capital gains and estate taxes, liberalize individual retirement accounts (IRAs), pull
the plug on welfare and the earned income tax credit (EITC),
and other such proposals that are guaranteed to widen the income gulf. The modest increase in the minimum wage accomplished near the end of President Clinton's first term stands
virtually as the sole exception that proves the rule.

Perhaps the answer to our puzzling national apathy toward

FIGURE 1.3

INCOME INEQUALITY IN
22 INDUSTRIALIZED COUNTRIES

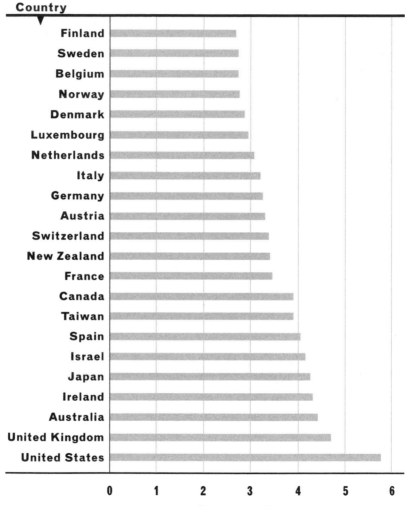

DECILE RATIO
(see text for explanation)

Source: Smeeding

inequality lies in our cultural predilection to admire economic freedom and individual opportunity. We shall return in a later chapter to the question of American attitudes toward opportunity and tolerance of inequality. Meantime, so long as the stock market continues to recover, and the economic gains of recent years protected, everyone has a crack at achieving the American Dream. But what is the evidence that we have, in fact, achieved the American Dream—"Life, liberty, and the pursuit of happiness"? Are we any happier today as a result of increased prosperity?

CHAPTER TWO

PROSPERITY AND HAPPINESS

DOES MONEY BUY HAPPINESS?

Writing thirty years ago, the skeptical economist E. J. Mishan mused about the prospects that rising affluence would deliver us from our wants:

> As we become richer, surely we shall remedy all social evils; heal the sick, comfort the aged and exhilarate the young. One has only to think with sublime credulity of the opportunities to be opened to us by the harvest of increasing wealth: universal adult education, free art and entertainment, frequent visits to the moon, a domesticated robot in every home and, therefore, woman forever freed from drudgery; for the common man, a lifetime of leisure to pursue culture and pleasure (or, rather, to absorb them from the TV screen); for the scientists, ample funds to devise increasingly powerful and ingenious computers so that we may

have yet more time for culture and pleasure and scientific discovery. . . . Here, then, is the panacea to be held with fervor. . . . What conceivable alternative could there be to economic growth? (Mishan, 1969, p. 4).

Looking back on the living standards that our parents enjoyed, and comparing them with where we stand today, many of us may question whether the rising affluence of the last thirty years has brought us "freedom from drudgery," "a lifetime of leisure to pursue culture," and the elimination of sickness and of all social evils.

If prosperity is supposed to have given us what we want, we ought to be deliriously happy by now. But what is the actual evidence that our economic performance resulted in increased stocks of happiness? Before we answer that question, we should address a few remarks about how we actually go about measuring happiness. Psychological investigations of happiness begin with assessments of subjective well-being (SWB). Researchers, for example, ask people to reflect on their happiness and life satisfaction with questions like, "How satisfied are you with your life as a whole these days? Are you very satisfied? satisfied? not very satisfied? not at all satisfied?" (Myers and Diener, 1995). It turns out that even such simple assessments can be relatively stable and reproducible over time, and correlate in the expected direction with other indicators of psychological well-being.

Searching for the sources of happiness has become something of a cottage industry in psychology. From what psychologists have so far uncovered, we know that a person's age, sex, and ethnic background provides very little clue about their levels of subjective well-being (Diener and Diener, 1998). On the other hand, having a supportive network of close relationships or being engaged by work and leisure, all seem to predict higher levels of happiness. What about having lots of money? Is the level of national wealth connected to stocks of happiness? Across nations of the world, it looks like per capita income predicts the level of happiness: The wealthier the country, the higher the average level of happiness among citizens (with a

FIGURE 2.1

MEAN LIFE SATISFACTION BY LEVEL OF ECONOMIC DEVELOPMENT

$r = .67$

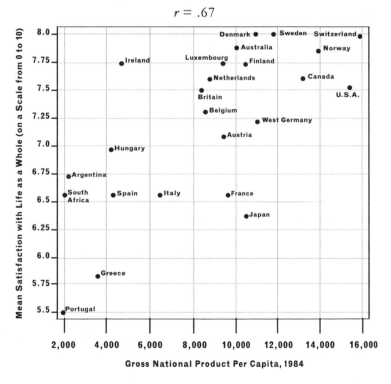

Gross National Product Per Capita, 1984

Source: Inglehart

correlation of about +0.67 in Figure 2.1). Americans are happier, on average, than citizens of Ethiopia. So far so good.

Paradoxically, though, there turns out to be only a weak relationship *within* industrialized countries between increasing income and levels of happiness. In very poor countries such as Bangladesh and India, personal income has been found to moderately predict levels of happiness, reflecting the fact that having access to food, shelter, and clothing is basic to well-being (Myers and Diener, 1995). In the case of such indigent countries, we conclude that having sufficient purchasing power to afford the basic needs of survival is an indispensable ingredient for the attainment of happiness. But what is the relevance of money for happiness in developed countries? Once people are able to afford life's basic necessities, it appears that further increases in the level of affluence matter rather little. Within the United States, Diener, et al. (1993), found a mere +0.12 correlation between personal income and happiness: Increases or decreases in income had no long-term influence on subjective well-being.

The evidence on the relationship between wealth and happiness over time is similarly unimpressive. In the U.S.A. real incomes rose substantially between 1940 and 1970, yet happiness seems to have peaked in the 1950s and then declined. In 1957, 35 percent of U.S. citizens polled told the National Opinion Research Center that they were very happy. In 1993, after incomes doubled, 32 percent said the same (Myers and Diener, 1995). Our level of national well-being has steadily diverged from the trajectory of rising prosperity (Figure 2.2).

Similarly, a study of Japan found no increase in subjective well-being from 1964 to 1981, despite the fact that real per capita GDP more than doubled (Easterlin, 1997). Noting that affluence gives little boost to human morale, a growing number of

FIGURE 2.2

HAPPINESS AND
ECONOMIC GROWTH IN THE U.S.A.

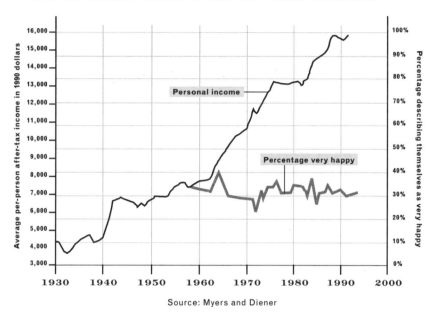

Source: Myers and Diener

psychologists have begun to speculate that perhaps people's
level of happiness depends not only on their own level of income, but on everyone else's. If everyone's income rises at the
same rate, it need not make anyone happier, since one's own
gains are offset by everyone else's success. But if this is true, then
the surge in income inequality during the past twenty years
should have given a dramatic boost to rich people's levels of happiness relative to the rest of society. Contrary to this conjecture,
people on *Forbes'* list of wealthiest Americans reported only
slightly greater happiness than other Americans. Indeed 37 percent owned that they were even less happy than the average
American (Diener et al., 1985). Similarly, a survey of twenty-two

major lottery winners revealed that they were no happier than a matched group of fellow Americans (Brickman, et al., 1978).

Could it be that affluence and happiness are unrelated because people adapt to their situation? After all, even the euphoria associated with winning the lottery wears off after a few months (Brickman, et al., 1978). Rising incomes generate rising expectations, and people quickly become accustomed to the new standard of living. The income requirement for fulfilling one's dreams is constantly revised upward with the changing standard of living. Material possessions beget the desire for even more possessions. Consider the case of the eighteenth-century philosopher Denis Diderot, whose parable, *Regrets on Parting with My Old Dressing Gown,* is retold in a recent book by the economist Juliet Schor:

> Diderot's regrets were prompted by a gift of a beautiful scarlet dressing gown. But in a short time, his pleasure turned sour as he began to sense that the surroundings within which the gown was worn did not properly reflect the garment's elegance. He grew dissatisfied with his study, with its threadbare tapestry, the desk, his chairs, and even the room's bookshelves. One by one, the familiar but well-worn furnishings of the study were replaced. In the end, Diderot found himself seated uncomfortably in the stylish formality of his new surroundings, regretting the work of this "imperious scarlet robe [that] forced everything else to conform with its own elegant tone" (Schor, 1998, p. 145).

As an illustration of the "Diderot effect," Schor (1998) found that Americans within every stratum of income were dissatisfied with what they earned. Sixty-four percent of Americans earning less than $10,000 per year responded in a survey that they "could not afford to buy everything they need." The unexpected finding was that in the same survey, 42 percent of Americans earning between $50,000 and $75,000 said the same, as well as 39 percent of Americans earning $75,000 to $100,000. In 1987, when the Roper polling organization asked Americans how much income per year they would need to fulfill their dreams, the median answer was $50,000. A few years later, in 1994, the median response had doubled, to $102,000. Moreover, the more affluent the respondent, the more money they said they needed to fulfill their American Dream. Thus, among those making more than $75,000, nearly two-thirds said they needed an increase of 50 to 100 percent in their annual income to be satisfied, while fewer than 20 percent of those making $30,000 or less said they needed as much (Schor, 1998).

If it is true that people's level of happiness depends upon their *expectations* based on past incomes, this would indeed tend to reduce the satisfaction that the rich obtain from their large incomes, whilst increasing the satisfaction that the poor derive from their meager incomes. But if the measurement of happiness depends on individuals' expectations and aspirations, this poses serious problems for using happiness as a yardstick of social welfare (more on this in a moment).

On the other hand, if happiness is contingent on "keeping up with the Joneses," as the evidence seems to suggest, then we would expect an individual's level of happiness to depend not just on what they make, but on what everybody else earns. This is in fact what Michael Hagerty, at the University of California, Davis, set out to test. Using data from the General Social Surveys, Hagerty looked at the correlation between levels of happiness and the degree of skew in the income distribution of 311 different communities across the United States (Hagerty, 2000). In line with theory, the higher the maximum income within a community, the less happy were residents at any given level of personal income. As the skew in the income distribution became more positive (i.e., the *fewer* rich individuals in a community), levels of happiness correspondingly increased. Tellingly, there was no relationship between the average level of income in a community versus individual levels of happiness—what mattered was the *distribution* of income, not the absolute level. Herein lies a possible explanation for the stagnation of national happiness in the United States since the 1970s. Because the distribution of incomes became more unequal during the same period that *average* incomes increased, the deleterious effects of the former on happiness canceled out any gains due to the latter trend. By contrast, several European countries that managed to keep a tighter rein on income inequality successfully increased average levels of happiness (Hagerty, 2000).

In less developed countries, the standard of living required to boost happiness now appears to be set by the wealthiest nations, because of the reach and influence of global communications. Ed Diener (2000), from the University of Illinois at Urbana–Champaign, has speculated that:

> People in China, India, and Nigeria want cars, refrigerators, VCRs, and the other possessions that they see on television. In other words, it may be that most people around the world now want many of the things that people in the West possess, and their life satisfaction is influenced to some degree by whether they are making progress toward obtaining these goods. Overall, increases in income in the wealthiest nations, however, do not raise levels of subjective well-being because

it is the rising living standards in these nations that influences people's level of desires. As income increases in the wealthiest nations, so does the evaluative standard (Diener, 2000, p. 39).

Recent evidence paints an even grimmer picture of the situation, where psychologists have discovered that merely *wishing* for more money seems to lead to unhappiness. Psychologists Tim Kasser and Richard Ryan (1996) distinguished between two classes of life goals. Individuals who valued and strove for financial success, fame, recognition, and good looks were categorized as having an *extrinsic* goal orientation, i.e., the satisfaction derived from attaining goals that depended on the approval and admiration of others. By contrast, individuals were classified as having an *intrinsic* goal orientation if they valued and sought personal growth through satisfying relationships with family and friends, and improving the world through activism. Such goals are called intrinsic in the sense of being inherently satisfying or valuable to the individual, rather than being dependent on the contingent evaluation of others. Among college students and adults, those who aspired toward extrinsic goals were significantly more likely to be depressed, to report experiencing fewer happy and joyful feelings, and more likely to report illness symptoms like headaches or malaise. Furthermore, such individuals were more likely to engage in destructive and nonproductive behaviors like cigarette smoking and watching television. In short, striving after fame and fortune should come with a government health warning: Chasing the American Dream can be hazardous to your well-being. Sadly, as Mihaly Csikszentmihalyi (1999) has pointed out, too many institutions in American society have a "vested interest in making people believe that buying the right car, the right soft drink, the right watch, the right education will vastly improve their chances of being happy, even if doing so will mortgage their lives."

WHY HAPPINESS IS NOT ENOUGH

While happiness is an intrinsic part of well-being, it is not sufficient by itself. Nearly everyone, no matter how destitute, finds some reason to feel cheerful at times. It is a part of the human survival instinct to respond to adversity, as illustrated by the seventeenth-century writer Thomas Browne: "I am the happiest man alive. I have that in me that can convert poverty into riches, adversity into prosperity, and I am more invulnerable than Achilles; fortune hath not one place to hit me." But the capacity of humans to adapt to the direst life circumstances should make us wary of using happiness as a gauge of social progress. As Amartya Sen observed:

> A thoroughly deprived person, leading a very reduced life, might not appear to be badly off in terms of the mental metric of desire and its fulfillment, if the hardship is accepted with non-grumbling resignation. In situations of long-standing deprivation, the victims do not go on grieving and lamenting all the time, and very often make great efforts to take pleasure in small mercies and to cut down personal desires to modest—"realistic"—proportions. Indeed, in situations of adversity which the individuals cannot individually change, prudential reasoning would suggest that the victims should concentrate their desires on those limited things that they *can* possibly achieve, rather than fruitlessly pining for what is unattainable. The extent of a person's deprivation,

then, may not at all show up in the metric of desire-fulfillment, even though he or she may be quite unable to be adequately nourished, decently clothed, minimally educated, and properly sheltered (Sen, 1992, p. 55).

The satisfaction generated by a good (e.g., food) is thus a woefully inadequate indicator of the welfare of an individual or a community. Utility (and, for that matter, happiness) is a mental indicator that is incapable of fully revealing certain effects. For example, the effects of malnutrition are not always perceived by the individual; one may take pleasure in a single crust of bread, but the lack of certain fundamental nutrients may scar one's body for life. There are, in fact, nonpsychological aspects of goods that are central to evaluating their advantages to people and society. Goods have characteristics that people may use to perform certain *functionings,* and it is the achievement of these functionings (being well-nourished, healthy, able to move, having self-respect, being respected, being able to take part in the life and progress of the community, and so forth) that indicates the benefit enjoyed by people (Acocella, 1998).

The achievement of society can obviously be evaluated in different ways, e.g., by the level of utility (such as the level of happiness), or by opulence (such as the volume and pleasure we derive from what we consume), or by the quality of life (such as our ability to function in valued ways) (Sen, 1992). Depending on which yardstick we pick, one may arrive at dramatically different judgments about the extent of progress achieved by a given society. For the neo-Aristotelian philosopher Martha Nussbaum, the proper yardstick of social welfare is the *capability* to perform valuable human functions or activities. Nussbaum's list of valuable capabilities fall into three categories: bodily

virtues (good health, nourishment, escaping avoidable morbidity and premature mortality); individuality virtues (ability to
have pleasurable experiences, function cognitively, make au-
tonomous choices, enjoy self-respect); and social virtues (ability
to engage in friendship, recreation, participation in family, communal, and political life). According to this framework, well-
being is defined by one's functionings in the bodily, individual,
and social domains, as well as the capabilities to perform those
activities (Crocker, 1997). Sen and Nussbaum's capability approach may be contrasted to welfarism in general and utilitari-
anism in particular, which sees value only in individual utility,
defined in terms of some mental characteristics, such as happiness, pleasure, or desire.

The capability approach departs from yet another commonly
adopted approach to social evaluation, namely per capita gross
national product (GNP). The world has become quite accustomed to comparing the performance of countries by the use of
GNP statistics. When the World Bank releases its annual league
table of GNP figures across the world, the leaders of countries
want to know if they are going up, or staying the same, and
where they stand in relation to others. But is national income a
good basis for evaluating achievement? Amartya Sen points out
that income is concerned with the *instruments* of achieving well-
being and other objectives, whereas the capability approach
views certain "doings and beings" (functionings) as important
and valuable in themselves.

To illustrate the distinction between judging social welfare by
the use of a yardstick such as "per capita GNP" with the capability approach, Sen (1992) demonstrates how the two can often
diverge in a spectacular way. Some of the most important forms
of functioning must surely include the elementary one of being

able to live long and avoid premature mortality—without it, one could hardly engage in other virtues such as participating in the life of the community. Evaluated in terms of per capita GNP, South Africa ($3,160), Gabon ($3,490), and Brazil ($3,640) have five to thirteen times the per capita GNP of Vietnam ($240), China ($620), and Sri Lanka ($700). Yet these comparatively wealthier countries provide their citizens with a significantly lower ability to survive premature mortality (with life expectancies varying between 54.5 and 66.6 years) than do the three lower-income countries (life expectancy range: 66.4 to 72.5 years) (Figure 2.3).

Costa Rica (GNP $2,610), which is also considerably poorer than South Africa, Gabon, or Brazil, offers not only a much higher life expectancy than those three (76.6 years), but a life expectancy that is not significantly below those in the richest countries of Europe and North America (with ten or more times Costa Rica's GNP per head). For example, the U.S.A., with a GNP per head of $26,980, has a life expectancy at birth of 76.4 years, whereas Costa Rica with a GNP per head of only $2,610 has already achieved a life expectancy of 76.6 years (Sen, 1992; UNDP, 1998). We shall return in a later section of the book to some potential explanations for the achievement of societies like China, Sri Lanka, and Costa Rica. The point that Sen is trying to make is that since income is not the sum total of human lives, the lack of money cannot be the sum total of human deprivation (UNDP, 1998). We may be happy, but suffer from a truncated span of life (or, for that matter, we may have excellent health status but feel dissatisfied).

We are not arguing for the substitution of health status as the only basis for evaluating societal achievement. Good health is certainly one of the goals that individuals value, but it is not (as

FIGURE 2.3

GNP PER CAPITA VS. LIFE EXPECTANCY

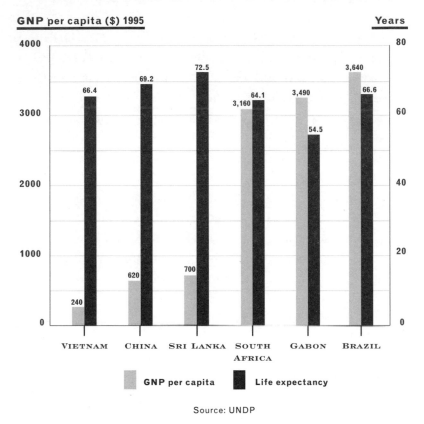

GNP per capita ($) 1995 — Years

Source: UNDP

some would claim) the only goal; the pursuit of health may sometimes even conflict with other goals. On the other hand, good health is an indispensable (and measurable) ingredient of an individual's capability set. We value health because of the freedom it provides us to pursue other plans and projects that we have reason to value. As Sen (1998) succinctly stated: "The dead cannot do much."

CHAPTER THREE

PROSPERITY
AND HEALTH

THE HEALTH OF NATIONS

Prosperity, we argued in the last chapter, does not buy happiness. The absence of money can breed misery, but having it is no guarantee of happiness. Happiness is thus a poor yardstick by which to judge social welfare. On the other hand, we made the case that good health is one of those essential ingredients of an individual's "capability set" that enables us to pursue the goals we value. What, then, is the evidence that money buys good health? Comparing countries across the world, there is no doubt that being poor is associated with reduced life expectancy. In Ethiopia, where we were introduced to the Getu family, the average life expectancy is fifty years for women, forty-seven years for men. In Mexico, where the average income is twenty-four times as high as Ethiopia, life expectancy is seventy-five years for women and sixty-nine years for men. And in the United States, home of the Skeen family, and one of the richest nations in the world, life expectancy is eighty years for women, seventy-three years for men (UNDP, 1998). To be sure, there are some countries in the world that have achieved an exceptionally high level of health in spite of being poor (Costa Rica was mentioned as an example in the previous chapter), and conversely, there are other countries that are underachievers despite being wealthy. But by and large, prosperity makes people live longer (Figure 3.1).

The link between prosperity and health undoubtedly reflects the kinds of things that money can buy: freedom from hunger,

FIGURE 3.1

RELATIONSHIP BETWEEN COUNTRY WEALTH AND LIFE EXPECTANCY

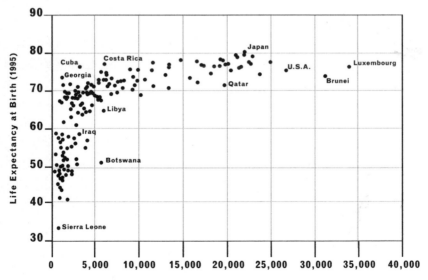

Per Capita Gross Domestic Product
(1995 U.S. $ purchasing power parties)

Source: UNDP

clean water supply, better sanitation, childhood immunization, access to medical technology, and so on. The same wealth fails to secure more happiness, presumably because human wants are insatiable, and people are forever chasing after goalposts that keep shifting with the rising material standard of living. Unlike happiness, however, the requirements for maintaining good health are finite and do not keep rising with the level of economic development. In fact, it takes rather little in the way of food, warmth, and shelter to fulfill basic human needs and maintain the organism in good shape. As we argued in the previous chapter, some of the principal threats to the health of people in affluent societies consist of excess consumption of one kind or another—too many calories in the diet, too much consumption of red meat, heavy drinking and smoking, and so on.

The observation that basic health needs are finite suggests that money will buy better health, but only up to a point. That is precisely the pattern observed in Figure 3.1. Up to a level of national income of about $5,000 per head (in 1990 U.S. dollars), there is a steep linear relationship between money and higher life expectancy. Beyond that point, however, further growth does not produce more health, and the relationship between income and life expectancy flattens out (Wilkinson, 1994). In spite of being the richest citizens on the globe, Americans do not enjoy the highest longevity in the world. Across twenty-eight OECD countries* in 1996, the range of life expectancies at birth ranged from a high of 83.6 years for Japanese women to a low of 65.9 years for Turkish men. If the level of affluence

* That is, countries belonging to the Organization for Economic Cooperation and Development (OECD).

is the main determinant of health, we would expect Americans to rank near the top of this list. Far from being the healthiest people in the world, American men ranked twenty-second out of twenty-eight OECD countries for life expectancy in 1996, while American women ranked nineteenth (Figures 3.2 A and B).

In terms of potential years of life lost due to premature mortality, Americans again ranked near the bottom (twenty-third and twenty-fourth, respectively, for men and women) out of twenty-eight OECD nations. As for infant mortality, the only nations in the OECD with a more dismal record than ours in 1996 were Turkey, Mexico, Hungary, Poland, and Korea (Anderson and Poullier, 1999). According to another comparison across thirteen large industrialized countries, the only health indicators on which the U.S. ranked comparatively favorably were life expectancy at age sixty-five (where Americans were seventh) and life expectancy at age eighty (where we ranked third) (Starfield, 1998).

Many Americans express surprise and dismay on discovering that life expectancy is higher in poorer countries like Greece, Spain, and Costa Rica, especially given that we spend by far the greatest amount on medical care—about $3,925 per capita compared with the OECD average of $1,728. What could account for our anomalous position? If money does not purchase more health beyond the threshold of meeting basic needs, then what does?

The economic historian and epidemiologist Richard Wilkinson has argued that once societies pass beyond the threshold of absolute deprivation, further increases in the size of the economic pie are not what matter for health achievement; it is how the slices of the pie are divided across society (Wilkinson, 1994;

FIGURE 3.2A

MEN'S LIFE EXPECTANCY

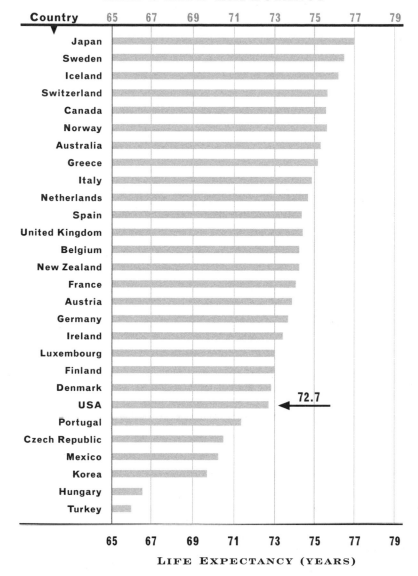

LIFE EXPECTANCY (YEARS)

Source: Anderson and Poullier

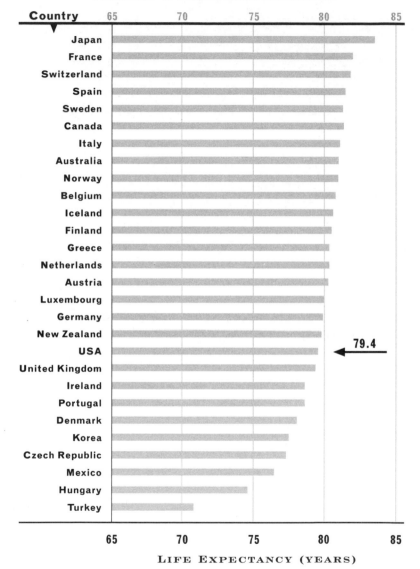

FIGURE 3.2B

WOMEN'S LIFE EXPECTANCY

LIFE EXPECTANCY (YEARS)

Source: Anderson and Poullier

1996). Wilkinson bases his conjecture on a comparison of data across OECD countries, which indicate a strong correlation between the distribution of income and life expectancy: The greater the inequality in the share of incomes, the lower the average life expectancy of that society (Wilkinson, 1986; 1992). The degree of income inequality in society explains about three-quarters of the variation in life expectancy across countries; whereas, by itself, the absolute size of the economic pie (measured by per capita GNP) accounts for less than 10 percent of the variation (Wilkinson, 1992). The implications of Wilkinson's theory for economic goals could hardly be more radical: If people wish to lead longer and healthier lives, then their governments had better start paying attention to a fairer distribution of the national product. Bigger is not necessarily better, when it comes to economic strategies for delivering longevity.

Wilkinson's original findings on OECD countries have been challenged by more recent data, which do not support a relationship between income distribution and life expectancy (Judge, 1995). However, his theory does not exclusively depend on the validity of data from industrialized countries (Kawachi, et al., 1999b). For example, several other studies based on less-developed countries (Rodgers, 1979; Flegg, 1982; Waldman, 1992; Wennemo, 1993) have examined the relationship between the distribution of income and infant mortality rates. These studies found that countries with unequal income distribution have higher rates of infant mortality than countries with similar levels of national product per capita but more equal income distributions. At first blush, this result may seem self-evident. After all, deaths among infants tend to occur more frequently among the poor, so that an unequal distribution of income may simply reflect the fact that there are more poor people in such societies, resulting in a higher average infant mortality rate. What is surprising, however, is that infant mortality appears to be positively correlated to the income share of the rich (the top 5 percent of the income distribution) when the incomes of the poor (the bottom 20 percent) are held constant among countries. Examining the relationship of income distribution to infant mortality rates across fifty-seven countries in 1960 and 1970, Waldman (1992) calculated that a 1 percent increase in the income share of the rich (while holding the share of other groups constant) was associated with an excess infant mortality rate of between 0.39 and 2.28 deaths per thousand live births, over and above the mean international rate of 53.8 deaths per thousand. This is a puzzling result, because an increase in the share of incomes of the rich while holding constant the share of poor people leaves their command over resources unchanged. So why should such an increase be associated with worse health outcomes among the poor?

Waldman (1992) examined a variety of potential explanations, such as differences in the relative accessibility of medical services associated with increased income inequality, lower female literacy rates, the degree of urbanization, increased fertility of the poor, and differences in the composition of births among different income groups. Despite carefully taking each of these variables into account, the association between infant mortality and the income share going to the rich remained positive and refused to go away.

THE RELATIVE INCOME HYPOTHESIS

Why, then, should the distribution of income matter for people's health, rather than their absolute level of income?

After considering (and rejecting) other possible explanations for the pattern of infant mortality across the world, Waldman conjectured that higher incomes for the rich led to a decline in breast feeding and a switch to bottle feeding. In turn, the behaviors of the rich may have distorted the preferences and judgments of the poor. The possibility that a poor person's level of well-being depends not just on their own income but on the levels of income (and behaviors) of others in society challenges conventional economic assumptions involved in making welfare comparisons. To use technical jargon, economists often resort to semi-Pareto conditions in making welfare comparisons: A country must be better off if every group receives a higher income than the comparable group in another country. However, if human welfare depends not just on one's own income but on the incomes of others in society, then results like Waldman's imply that the absolute standard of living may be a poor measure of social welfare: When incomes are unequally distributed, the true welfare of the poor may be lower than measured income suggests (Waldman, 1992).

The significance of people's relative income is more far-reaching than the example of infant mortality suggests—low social status and the accompanying sense of relative deprivation have been shown to produce physiological responses in individuals that may damage their health in multiple ways. We shall discuss later the variety of evidence that suggests that relative deprivation—being lower on the social ladder—is harmful to health. For the moment, let us critically examine the assumption that an individual's welfare is determined solely by the absolute quantities of various goods she consumes, not on how those quantities compare with the amounts consumed by others around her.

A good deal of evidence suggests that people pay attention to their *relative* position in society. Economists Sara Solnick and David Hemenway recently carried out a survey of graduate students and faculty at the Harvard School of Public Health, asking them to make a series of choices between two hypothetical worlds (Solnick and Hemenway, 1998). For example, respondents were asked to pick which of the two worlds they preferred to live in:

A. Your current yearly income is $50,000; others earn $25,000.
B. Your current yearly income is $100,000; others earn $250,000. (Assume that the purchasing power of money is the same in states A and B).

Given the choice between these two hypothetical worlds, *homo economicus* would have no hesitation about choosing the latter. After all, you would be twice as well off in the second world. The choice, in conventional economics terms, is what would be called a no-brainer.

However, many readers may disagree with this response, preferring to live in a world where others earn less, even if it means they themselves would earn less. Nor would they be alone in making this judgment. As Solnick and Hemenway discovered, fully 56 percent of their subjects preferred the world in which they earned less in absolute terms but more in relative terms. The same kinds of preferences were also expressed for numbers of years of education. Given the following choice:

A. You have twelve years of education (high school); others have eight.

B. You have sixteen years of education (college); others
    have twenty (graduate degree).

Half of the respondents preferred the former. About the only
area in which respondents were insensitive to what everyone
else had was the amount of vacation time. Apparently, almost
everyone would prefer more leisure regardless of how much
everyone else was getting. In their informal comments after
completing the survey, respondents volunteered that their
choices were not motivated primarily by envy. As Solnick and
Hemenway reported:

> Many seemed to see life as an ongoing competition, in which
> not being ahead means falling behind. In their view, consis-
> tent with theorists who emphasize the instrumental nature
> of positional concerns, a higher relative standing leads to
> such desirable outcomes as access to better jobs and edu-
> cation, improved marital prospects and the opportunity to
> pass these advantages to one's children (Solnick and
> Hemenway, 1998, p. 379).

In other words, having less is sometimes more. Instead of
leveling accusations of envy and irrationality at noneconomists
who express such preferences, the economics profession might
serve policy better by reconsidering their assumptions.

Some famous studies conducted in the U.S. military during
the 1940s echo this point. Researchers found that morale was
actually higher among officers in the military police, where promotion rates were very *slow*, compared with officers in the air
force, where promotion was very rapid (Stouffer, et al., 1949;
Merton and Rossi, 1950). This paradoxical finding was appar-

ently due to the sense of relative deprivation experienced by the large number of officers in the air force who were promoted less rapidly than the few who were successful. The conjecture that a person's level of well-being depends not just on their own level of income, but on everybody else's, is referred to as "the relative income hypothesis." People pay a lot more attention to relative standing than economists might assume.

POVERTY AS A RELATIVE CONCEPT

Additional evidence of the relative framework by which we judge the world derives from the way people think of poverty. Since 1965, the U.S. government has defined poverty according to absolute criteria. Based on Mollie Orshansky's work at the Social Security Administration, the U.S. official poverty line was determined on the basis of the cost of a minimum diet needed to feed an average poor family, with an adjustment to allow for other needed expenses, such as housing and clothing. The diet itself—the Economy Food Plan, as it was called—was put together by the U.S. Department of Agriculture by surveying the food-buying patterns of low-income families in 1955 as well as their nutritional requirements. The Food Plan was designed for "temporary or emergency use when funds were low," and allowed for no eating at restaurants, called for careful management of food storage and preparation, and was acknowledged at the time to provide a nutritious though monotonous diet. Except for minor modifications since its official adoption by the federal government in 1965, the definition of the poverty line has remained unchanged. Each year, the threshold is updated for inflation using the Consumer Price Index—but overall, we

continue to define poverty based on the minimum food requirements of a poor family in the 1950s (Citro and Michael, 1995).

In stark contrast to the way that federal government defines
poverty, representative opinion polls of the American public
consistently suggest that people define poverty in relative terms.
Thus, based on evidence from the Gallup Poll conducted over
the last three decades, it is apparent that the American public defines poverty as a level of income that is less than half of the
median family income. Figure 3.3, from the National Research

FIGURE 3.3

ALTERNATIVE POVERTY THRESHOLDS
FOR FOUR-PERSON FAMILIES
IN CONSTANT 1992 DOLLARS

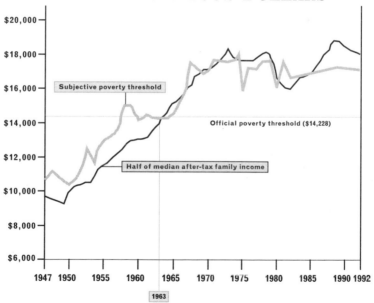

Source: Citro and Michael

Council's 1995 report on measuring poverty, compares the official poverty threshold to popular opinion about where the cut-off should lie (Citro and Michael, 1995).

Whereas the official poverty line has remained flat since 1965 (after adjustment for inflation), the Gallup Poll definition of the poverty line has steadily risen during the last three decades, indicating that people's notions about what constitutes poverty is revised upward in line with rising societal living standards. The only time that the subjective poverty threshold agreed with the official threshold was, in fact, back in 1965 when the federal government adopted its current definition. The two lines have steadily diverged since. When we plot the trend line for "half the median family income," there turns out to be good agreement between that graph and the subjective poverty threshold. Notably, during periods of economic recession (when real incomes fell), people's subjective judgments about the poverty threshold also falls in tandem. Over the long haul, as the average incomes of Americans have risen in real terms, so too have popular conceptions of how much money it takes to stay out of "being poor." People judge the world in relative terms. Needless to add, successive administrations have shown reluctance to adopt the relative definition of poverty, because doing so would result in an overnight jump in the number of Americans living in poverty, even if it reflects the reality of people's perceptions.

The relative income hypothesis is a powerful critique of the "trickle-down" theory of economic growth, which maintains that societal welfare can be increased by focusing on economic policies that raise everyone's incomes, without regard for distributional concerns. This might be true in societies that have not yet reached the level of development necessary to satisfy basic needs such as adequate nutrition or shelter. However, among societies that have passed that threshold, the relative income hypothesis predicts that (for example) doubling everyone's standard of living without altering the underlying distribution of resources will not necessarily result in improvements in the average level of well-being. It is not sufficient that everyone's incomes are rising by a certain amount. What matters is the distance between the rich and the poor in society. Most Americans living in poverty still have access to indoor plumbing, electricity, heat, a television set, and perhaps an old car. In many less-developed countries, the American poor would be considered rich. Yet the poor in America feel poor simply because their reference group consists of other Americans living around them, and in relation to this group they are poor. As society becomes more prosperous, the definition of what constitutes poverty has to be revised upward (Blumberg, 1980).

A corollary of the relative income hypothesis is that, if people's health is responsive to their relative position in society, then one would expect to observe differences in well-being *within* societies comparing individuals with more or less income relative to others (Wilkinson, 1997). This is exactly the pattern that has been reported in study after study within different countries (Adler, et al., 1994). Even though there is no relationship between aggregate income and life expectancy *across* industrialized countries, differences have been found in the health status of individuals *within* societies according to their relative position in the economic hierarchy. (The apparent paradox that income differences *between* rich countries don't predict health status, whereas income difference *within* them do, presumably has to do with the relevant units of social comparison: People compare themselves with others in their own society, but not to others outside national boundaries.)

Within societies, the lower our standing relative to others, the unhealthier we tend to be. For example, in the Panel Study of Income Dynamics, a nationally representative sample of American families, individuals whose household incomes were less than $15,000 (in 1993 dollars) were three times as likely to die of any cause during the study follow-up compared with individuals whose incomes were more than $70,000 (McDonough, et al., 1997) (Figure 3.4).

FIGURE 3.4

RELATIVE RISKS OF ALL-CAUSE MORTALITY BY HOUSEHOLD INCOME LEVEL

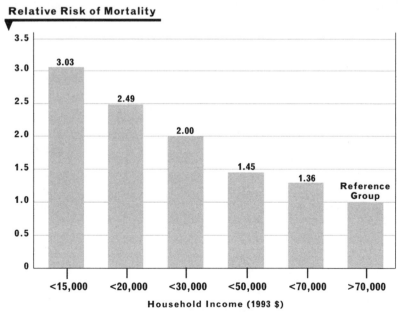

Source: McDonough, et al.

WHAT EXPLAINS SOCIOECONOMIC DIFFERENCES IN HEALTH?

It is tempting to attribute the poor health of individuals near the bottom of the economic ladder to the lack of access to material comforts enjoyed by the well-to-do. However, as we noted earlier, in an affluent society such as the United States, there are diminishingly few things that the poor cannot afford that would make a difference between life and death. For sure, there are serious shortfalls in essential consumption in this society—an estimated 30 million Americans, including 13 million children under twelve, are hungry because of difficulty getting the food they need (UNDP, 1998). However, the reality is that for most families in America now, the economic challenge is not to acquire the goods they *need* but the goods they *want*. For instance, in 1920, the bottom 20 percent of earners spent 70 percent of their incomes on basic necessities such as food, clothing, and shelter; but now that proportion is down to 45 percent (Frank, 1999; p. 15).

Readers may object that health care is very expensive in America, and that not being able to afford health insurance could make the difference between life and death for the 47 million uninsured and underinsured Americans. There is no doubt that lack of access to health care could make a huge difference to the course of life-threatening diseases like asthma, diabetes, hypertension, and heart disease. The poor are also denied access to screening and preventive services that could make the difference in terms of the early detection and treatment of cancer and a host of other serious conditions. There is no gainsaying that the health status of Americans is worse off as a result of the egregious inequalities in access to medical services. Nonetheless, lack of access to health care cannot be solely responsi-

ble for the pattern of health inequality (shown in figure 3.4), because exactly the same kinds of health inequalities by socioeconomic status are observed in countries like the United Kingdom
and Sweden, whose citizens have long enjoyed universal access
to health care (Kunst, 1997). Health care and medical technology can make the difference between life and death if you happen to be sick, but it is not the major explanation for why some
people get sick in the first place while others stay healthy. By the
time a middle-aged individual presents to the emergency room
with a heart attack, the damage done to his coronary arteries
represents the bodily injuries cumulated over a lifetime through
smoking habits initiated during adolescence, poor diet practiced
throughout adulthood, exposure to stressful jobs, and so on. In
other words, we need to look elsewhere to account for the socioeconomic gradient in health.

Another common explanation for health inequalities, partic-
ularly popular among economists, is that they reflect reverse
causation, i.e., ill health causes loss of income. There can be no
denying that illness causes loss of income due to both employment interruption (or even loss of employment), as well as the
extra medical costs attending illness. Such effects are doubly
crippling for poor people who lack the financial savings to tide
them over emergencies, and who can ill afford the medical costs
imposed by illness. In global terms, economists have come to
recognize that illness can have a major impact on productivity
and gross national product, especially among less-developed
countries ravaged by epidemics of diseases such as malaria and
HIV/AIDS (Bloom and Canning, 2000). So which comes first:
illness or poverty? Illness can certainly cause loss of income, but
interpreting the evidence in this way begs the question of what
causes some individuals to fall sick in the first place. Although

this riddle has the appearance of a "chicken or egg" problem, most experts now agree that the arrow of causation runs predominantly from low income to poor health, rather than the reverse. We know this because studies have tracked individuals from relatively early on in their careers (when they were free of illness), and demonstrated that low incomes lead to the higher onset of morbidity and premature mortality, rather than the other way round (Wilkinson, 1996).

So if it is not access to health care or reverse causation, what then accounts for the gradient in health shown in Figure 3.4? A third category of explanation is that the differences are due to the adoption of unhealthy "lifestyles" by the poor. Poor people, it is argued, suffer a greater burden of ill health because they choose to engage in unhealthy behaviors such as cigarette smoking, lack of exercise, fatty diets, and so on. While countless surveys have confirmed that such unhealthy behaviors are indeed more common among low-income people, it is surely myopic to rest the case with this argument. This is because many lifestyles that we now associate with the poor in economically developed countries were, in fact, more common among affluent individuals at an earlier stage in history. For instance, cigarette smoking and high red meat intake were both more common among the upper classes during earlier times in this country, because you needed the disposable income to be able to indulge in these "lifestyles." (Indeed, in many less-developed countries today, these habits remain confined to those who can afford them). Similarly, sedentary lifestyles and obesity used to be markers of what Veblen (1912) called "conspicuous leisure and consumption." For poor people toiling in the fields, or in heavy manual labor, obtaining the daily amount of physical activity recommended by the surgeon general to stay lean was not a matter of choice. The very fact that the pattern and distribution of "lifestyles" is historically contingent implies that we are dealing with superficial explanations of the gradient—or epiphenomena. In order to understand the reason for socioeconomic disparities in health, we must delve into deeper, more fundamental, causes.

So what is "it" that explains why being lower on the socioeconomic ladder is toxic for health? What could account for the difference in mortality risk between someone who makes $50,000 per year versus someone who makes $70,000 (Figure 3.4)? In the Panel Study of Income Dynamics, the poorest individuals had three times the risk of dying compared with the richest. Nevertheless, the risk did not stop there, but extended well into what we would consider the middle-class range of incomes, so that even individuals with household incomes in the $50,000 to 70,000 range experienced a 36 percent excess risk of death during the follow-up compared with the most affluent group (Figure 3.4). The difference in risk of death between someone earning $50,000 and someone making $70,000 cannot be due to the former class of individuals being unable to afford the basic necessities of life. Could the difference be due to access to luxury goods?

In Britain, not owning an automobile has been described as the "single most important indicator" of mortality risk (Davey Smith, et al., 1994). In the Office of National Statistics Longitudinal Study, a follow-up of a 1 percent sample from the British Census, mortality in 1981–89 was 41 percent higher for men and 24 percent higher for women in non–car owning households compared with those in car-owning households (Filatki and Fox, 1995). These differences persist within social class groups. Even among the top administrators in the famous

Whitehall Study of British civil servants, those without access to cars had higher mortality than those with cars (Davey Smith, et al., 1990). Yet what is it about car ownership that should make a difference to longevity? Consider as a thought experiment what would happen if the Getu family in Ethiopia suddenly won a '99 Honda Civic in a lottery: Would it dramatically improve their chances of longevity? The answer is not immediately obvious. Indeed, one can think of several aspects of car ownership that are damaging to health, such as the increased risk of being in a motor vehicle accident, or the increased risk of obesity due to a drop in levels of physical activity (Macintyre, et al., 1998). Why car ownership matters is not because of any absolute survival advantage it confers, but because not having a car can hurt a person's access to opportunities and resources in an economy where *everyone else drives a car*. Sociologist Christopher Jencks (1992) put it in the following way:

"In 1900 . . . America was organized on the assumption that city residents would get around on foot or by streetcar. Outside the cities, Americans traveled by foot or horse. In such a world an automobile was clearly a luxury. Over the course of the twentieth century, however, most Americans acquired cars. This had two effects. First, public transportation atrophied. Second, most employers and shops moved to areas that were accessible only by car, and most families did the same. Outside a few major cities, therefore, not having a car meant not being able to get to work, to shops, or to friends' homes, making a car a necessity for most Americans."

In other words, access to a car matters to health in affluent societies because it can determine access to employment, to

shops selling healthy foods at affordable prices, to leisure facilities, social support networks, and health services (Macintyre,
et al., 1998). Above all, in a society where car ownership is nearly
universal, not owning one (or not owning the latest model) begins to threaten an individual's sense of "ontological security,"
i.e., their sense of person-hood and prestige (Macintyre, et al.,
1998). These advantages would be hardly relevant in a society
where everyone went about on foot and few individuals drove
cars. Lack of access to a car is thus not so much a marker of life-
threatening hardship, but a rather sensitive indicator of *relative*
deprivation.

We have come full circle, then, to the relative income hypothesis as the most likely explanation for the socioeconomic differences in health demonstrated in Figure 3.4. Lacking income is
harmful to health because low income is an exquisite indicator
of one's *relative* position in society. "Low income" only has
meaning in reference to what others make in society. An annual
income of $10,000 is "low" in a society like the United States
where the average person earns $30,000. If the average income
suddenly doubled, the person earning $10,000 would be not
only a lot poorer but also a lot less healthy.

CHAPTER FOUR

KEEPING UP WITH THE [DOW] JONESES

PROSPERITY AND THE RISE OF CONSUMER SOCIETY

One of the consequences of economic growth, as we have just seen, has been to transform the material and social environment in ways that raise the real cost of living for most individuals in that society (Wilkinson, 1986). Many consumer goods have followed the same trajectory as the automobile, starting out as luxuries but gradually becoming necessities. As Sen (1992) describes it: "While the rural Indian may have little problem in appearing in public without shame with relatively modest clothing and can take part in the life of the community without a telephone or a television, the commodity requirements of these general functionings are much more demanding in a country where people standardly use a bigger basket of diverse commodities."

The dress code required in everyday American life is much

more demanding than in rural India. What suit should we wear for that crucial job interview? How should we dress for "casual Fridays" at the office? These seemingly trivial questions would seem to have little to do with the questions of economic necessity or survival noted earlier. So why do we agonize so much about what we wear? In obeying sartorial customs, we undergo distresses that are, from a strictly economic point of view, needless and futile. As Quentin Bell (1976) wryly observed: "We may protest against the tyranny of tailors and dressmakers; but their commands are continually urged upon us by our sense of propriety." The reason we care about community standards of dress is because once such conventions are established, being ill-dressed can make the difference between getting a job, obtaining credit, finding a mate, or simply avoiding adverse notice (especially from the police or security guards). Even if we choose to flout conventions, it is often the spouses, the friends, or our companions who can end up suffering the consequences of our rebellion.

Take another example: telephones were a luxury in 1900, when hardly anyone had one.

> But today, when almost everyone has a telephone, those without service are cut off from family and friends, who no longer write letters. Indeed, those without telephones often have trouble even keeping a job, both because employers now expect workers to call in if they are sick and because workers without telephones cannot make hasty changes in their child-care or transportation arrangements (Jencks, 1992).

Not having access to a telephone in American society is thus a major handicap and a constant source of stress, but mainly because everyone else owns one. The question for consumers these days is not whether to own one, but how many of them they should own (the average American household has three, including at least one cordless), and which models they should purchase. Rotary phones were an improvement on previous models when they first came out, but soon became unsatisfying when touch-tone phones appeared on the market. Indeed now that everyone owns a touch-tone telephone, one of the banes of our daily lives has become navigating the thicket of touch-tone instructions that are commonplace in the recorded messages of government departments, hospitals, commercial airlines, and even the complaints departments of retail businesses. Moreover, the once-humble household instrument has undergone a transformation to become a status symbol on its own. Gone are the days when the telephone just used to serve the utilitarian purpose of connecting distant people. No one seems content to opt for the $9.99 no-frills model anymore. The latest thing to have is the $249.99 model with the two-line cordless speakerphone and intercom, which comes with Caller ID and has a built-in answering machine and headset jack, a flash button for Call Waiting, plus keys for speed dialing, mute, hold, redial, and page (Hafner, 1999). Besides communicating with distant people, telephone owners use them now to communicate their material success to others.

The rise in ownership of various consumer commodities over the last thirty years is charted in Figure 4.1. From the figure, we can see that even back in 1970, most American homes (87 percent) were equipped with telephones, but by 1995, the proportion had risen to 93.7 percent. Several other consumer goods, such as the personal computer and the answering machine, were nonexistent in 1970, but have subsequently attained the status of virtual necessities (Figure 4.1).

FIGURE 4.1

THE RISING OWNERSHIP OF CONSUMER GOODS

(ADAPTED FROM COX AND ALM)

OWNERSHIP IN ITEM	1970	MID-1990's
Homes lacking a telephone[a]	13.0%	6.3%
Households with no vehicle[a]	20.4%	7.9%
Households with two or more vehicles[a]	29.3%	61.9%
Households with computer	0%	41.0%
Households with answering machine	0%	65.0%
Households with a microwave	<1%	89.5%
Households with color TV	34.0%	97.9%
Households with cable TV	6.3%	63.4%
Households with two or more TVs	30.7%	72.8%
Households with videocasette recorder	0%	89.0%
Households with frost-free refrigerator	<25%	86.8%
New homes with central heating and air conditioning	34.0%	81.0%

[a] Data for 1995. The rest are data for 1997.

The pattern of rising ownership of consumer goods can elicit quite different reactions about the performance of the American economy over the past three decades. Some find cause to celebrate the fact that Americans own more of everything in the 1990s than they did in 1970 (Cox and Alm, 1999). Yet others see in this same pattern cause for alarm about the increasing demands that consumer culture exerts on poor (and middle-class) families to keep up with the affluent, especially during an era of widening income inequalities (Schor, 1998).

The tendency for the American Dream to enlarge over time is clearly revealed in surveys of consumer wants and needs, documented by Juliet Schor (1998):

FIGURE 4.2

SURVEYS OF AMERICAN CONSUMPTION WANTS AND NEEDS (PERCENTAGE OF RESPONDENTS)

(FROM SCHOR, 1998)

	1975	1991	PERCENTAGE CHANGE
What makes a good life?			
Vacation home	19	35	+84
Swimming pool	14	19	+36
Jobs that pays more	45	60	+33
Interesting job	38	38	0
Happy marriage	84	77	− 8
What is a necessity?			
Second television	3	10	+233
Home air conditioning	26	51	+96

A notable trend during the past two decades has been the contrasting difference between the massive intensification of consumption wants for *material* goods, but the stagnation (or even decline) of expressed needs for spiritual goods, such as a fulfilling job or happy marriage. As we shall argue, these trends have dire implications for not only the happiness of Americans, but also their health and well-being.

The connection between rising prosperity and the intensification of consumer culture was presaged by the late economist Fred Hirsch, in his influential work, *Social Limits to Economic Growth* (1976). In his book, Hirsch distinguished between goods that meet our material needs and so-called "positional goods"—those that we value because others do not have them. So long as material privation is widespread, the conquest of material scarcity is the dominant concern of society, and the consumption habits of the majority of the population are concentrated on basic material goods. The positional sector of the economy is correspondingly small: In many of its aspects, the frontier of wants is still open. Positional competition is largely confined to the purely representational, to indications of relative superiority. As Hirsch pointed out, positional consumption may be socially resented in poor societies, but it is economically benign. Economists dating back to Adam Smith (1759) have observed that prosperous individuals in indigent societies are obliged by the inadequate capacities of their stomachs to sell their surplus by purchasing "those baubles and trinkets" that provide the means of support to others who supply their needs. Thus the rich are led in this way "by an invisible hand . . . and without intending it, without knowing it . . . [to] advance the interests of society." The rich could be encouraged to chase "trinkets" so long as this contributed to the wider good. For society, and especially for the poor, this exchange was plainly a good deal, as they reaped a correspondingly large consumer surplus.

However, as the wealth of a society increases, and material needs are met, the demand for former luxuries becomes more extensively diffused throughout the population. As the frontier of basic wants closes, demand for the acquisition of positional goods spreads and intensifies. Competition shifts increasingly from the material sector to the positional sector. And to the extent that particular positional goods become actively sought for the performance of specific functions beyond "representation"—for example, owning a car to gain access to jobs—the appurtenances of the rich cease to become "baubles and trinkets," and turn into squirrels' wheels for those below (Hirsch, 1976).

The process that Hirsch was describing is intimately linked to the rise of the modern consumer society. But where Hirsch saw an inevitable connection between economic growth and the rise of positional competition, our claim is that such competition is vastly exacerbated by patterns of economic growth that widen the gap between the rich and the rest of society. We may now state our proposition: that the greater the degree of income inequality in society, the more entrenched consumer culture becomes. Undoubtedly, as Hirsch claimed, economic growth alone will raise the commodity requirements of individuals striving to take part in the life of the community. But at the same time, the more unequal is the pattern of income growth across groups in society, the more unbalanced consumption patterns tend to be, and in turn, the more intense the competition for the acquisition of positional goods. What the wealthy have today cannot be delivered to the rest of us tomorrow: "yet as we individually grow richer, that is what we expect. . . . The intensified positional competition involves an increase in needs for the individual, in the sense that additional resources are required to achieve a given level of welfare" (Hirsch, 1976, p. 67).

Intense positional competition feeds consumer culture. The essential character of consumer society has been set forth by other writers: "A consumer society is one in which the possession and use of an increasing number and variety of goods and services is the principal cultural aspiration and the surest perceived route to personal happiness, social status, and national success" (Ekins, 1991); and "A consumer society makes the development of new consumer goods and the desire for them into a central dynamic of its socioeconomic life. An individual's self-respect and social esteem are strongly tied to his level of consumption relative to others in society" (Segal 1995).

It is surely no coincidence that American society, which tolerates the greatest disparities in wealth and incomes among industrialized countries, also leads the world in terms of the ferocity of its consumer culture (everyone must own bigger cars, more spacious homes, wider TV screens). The goods and services whose consumption characterizes a consumer society are not those that are needed for subsistence, but are "valued for non-utilitarian reasons, such as status seeking, envy provocation, and novelty seeking" (Goodwin, 1997). As anyone who has traveled to Western Europe cannot help but notice, more egalitarian societies there do not exhibit nearly the same level of consumerism. It is uncommon to see even wealthy Europeans driving about town in monstrous, gas-guzzling, four-wheel-drive sports utility vehicles. But the moment a traveler returns to the United States and steps off the plane, we are quickly reminded again of the consumption excesses in this country, whether it consists in the glimpses of overnourished and overweight Americans queuing in front of the airport doughnut or hot dog concession, or the armada of minivans, jeeps, and luxury pickup trucks that one must navigate through in order to get out of the car park. And as you drive out of the airport into the city, the ubiquitous signs of conspicuous consumption and conspicuous waste are made doubly poignant by the visible evidence of social exclusion in the form of homeless people on the streets.

A quick indicator of consumer culture is the number of words we use in everyday language to describe common objects. Inside the Arctic Circle, where there are few material things to acquire (but there is abundant snow), the Inuit culture has developed over forty words to describe the different types of snow. In impoverished Burkina Faso, the women have at least eight different words to describe the types of diarrhea that their infants routinely succumb to. Here in the United States, we employ dozens of different words to describe the types of automobiles: compact cars, convertibles, station wagons, minivans, sedans, SUVs, stretch limousines, and so on.

Yet another indicator of consumer culture is spending on luxury goods. Fed by the recent economic boom, firms producing luxury goods posted record sales and profits throughout the 1990s. True, the economic downturn of 2001, combined with the September 11 terrorist attacks, have dampened the consumer's appetite for ostentatious luxury. But that still did not stop Neiman Marcus from advertising its $6.7 million customized helicopter (with entertainment center) in its Christmas 2001 catalog, or the limited-edition jar of La Mer face cream for $1,200, or the $65 mink-covered coat hanger (Kaufman, 2001).

As a final example of an indicator of consumer culture, consider the amount that a society spends on advertising consumer products. It is no coincidence that the top ten countries in the world that spent the most in advertising as a proportion of their GDP in the mid-nineties include some of the most unequal societies in the world—such as Colombia, Brazil, Venezuela, Australia, New Zealand, the UK, and, of course, the United States

(UNDP, 1998). When we test the association between income inequality and advertising expenditure in a more formal manner, a striking association emerges. Figure 4.3 shows the correlation between a measure of income distribution (the decile ratio of household incomes introduced in figure 1.2 back in Chapter 1) and the percent of gross domestic product that each country in the Luxembourg Income Study spends on advertising.

The countries that spend the most lavishly on advertising also tend to be the most unequal—the U.S.A., UK, and Australia. The more unequal the income distribution, the greater the penetration of consumer culture, at least as measured by advertising expenditure (with a correlation coefficient of 0.68).

CRITIQUES OF THE CONSUMER CULTURE

Throughout history, societies have expressed disapproval of conspicuous consumption by passing various forms of sumptuary laws. For example, dating all the way back to Roman times, sumptuary laws forbade a wide range of expenditures that were deemed excessive, including the specification that funeral pyres should be made of unfinished, not polished wood (Frank, 1999). In medieval Florence, regulations limited the number of courses served during an evening meal, which restriction inspired the elaborate one-dish meals like the pastry-wrapped, meat-and-pasta torte (Frank, 1999). Similarly heavy-handed approaches to curbing consumer exuberance have been tried in different societies during different historical periods, but they all inevitably failed. Although modern consumer culture has also been criticized on moral grounds, it is not the frivolous nature of much of conspicuous consumption that we are con-

FIGURE 4.3

THE RELATIONSHIP OF INCOME INEQUALITY TO NATIONAL ADVERTISING EXPENDITURES

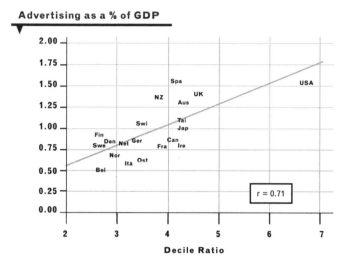

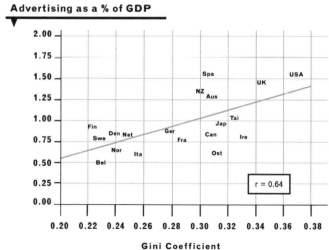

Source: Adapted from "Advertising Expenditure Forecasts"
(July 1999), prepared by Zenith Media (authors: Jonathan
Barnard, Kate Harrad, Adam Smith, and Steven Vass)

cerned about. What we really care about is when consumption patterns damage society through social exclusion, distortion of priorities in social investment, or contribute to the degradation of the social and physical environment. In short, a persuasive critique of the consumer society needs to focus on enumerating the *costs* of consumption. To quote the economist Juliet Schor (1997): we need to offer people "a more appealing version of an alternative society." Schor offers three positive (as opposed to normative) bases for the critique of consumer society, each of which we shall examine in some detail:

Firstly, the neoclassical economic model assumes that workers freely choose the hours they work, and consumers what they spend. In conventional economic analysis, therefore, whatever outcomes ensue from their choices are assumed to be optimal, in the sense that workers/consumers are "getting what they want." But if most workers cannot choose their hours of work, then there is no sense in which the current trade-off between leisure and income, or leisure and consumption, is optimal. The neoclassical presumption of worker/consumer sovereignty is undermined. Workers who are constrained to work more than they would choose, and become habituated to spending the resulting income, end up "wanting what they get."

Secondly, many goods and services are underpriced: They do not take account of costs imposed on others (what economists term "negative externalities")—for example, the increased traffic congestion, emission of greenhouse gases, and more serious accidents caused by the current fad for sports utility vehicles. In other words, there is "excess" consumption of goods and services compared with the optimal level that would exist in the absence of such external effects. Consumption clearly contributes to social welfare when it enriches the lives of people without affecting the well-being of others.

Thirdly, consumerism undermines community. The decline of free time outside the workplace diminishes opportunities to maintain community, friendship, and family ties. As we shall argue in a later chapter, declining community ties diminishes the health status of citizens. As we can see from Schor's list, the costs of consumer culture are tightly linked with the societal price we pay for income inequality. The more unequal the distribution of income, the longer and harder families need to work to keep from slipping behind on the economic ladder. The greater the disparities in wealth and income, the greater the effort expended by producers of goods and services in catering to the spending habits of the rich—more space on first-class seats in commercial airlines, building bigger cars and more spacious houses, and so on. As the consumption patterns of the rich become more normative, the more ordinary families need to spend to keep up with the average standard of living. The harder families work to pay for lifestyles beyond their means, the less time we invest in maintaining family and community ties. The more caught up we become in competitive spending, the less regard we have for the external costs our habits impose on the social and physical environment.

CONSUMER CULTURE AND CONSUMER DEBT

Fed by the income inequality that divides the population, American businesses have increasingly taken to targeting their products to households at the upper end of the income spectrum, those earning $50,000 or more (Uchitelle, 1997). And in turn, the consumption patterns of the rich have dragged everyone into a spending arms race. In an era of too much merchandise competing for buyers, companies long ago discovered that they cannot make a profit by simply raising prices for standard products. So they have taken to squeezing out profits by adding ever more gimmicks and embellishments to existing products, with which they hope to lure consumers to pay extra. Extra profits are embedded in each new gimmick—like all the extra jacks, buttons, and features that are built in to justify the $250 telephone set as opposed to the $10 model (it rings, you pick it up). Even companies that make low-priced goods for the less affluent have been tapping into the trend, counting on the easier spending of the affluent to rub off on lower-income households. For instance, Rubbermaid introduced an $18 water filter in the late 1990s to go with one of its plastic pitchers (Uchitelle, 1997).

Proceeding *pari passu* with the growth in luxury spending, "shopping disorder" has emerged as a new disease category, a form of addiction (Rozhon, 1998). According to David W. Krueger, a Houston psychiatrist who published a self-help book on diagnosing this disorder (*Emotional Business: The Meanings of Work, Money and Success,* Avant Books/Slawson Communications, 1992), the diagnostic hallmarks of this disorder include compulsive shopping, competitive shopping, and revenge shopping (spending a loved one's money to exact punishment). Many people shop to overcome feelings of loneliness. Or they shop in order to assuage their guilt about spending too much time at work and not enough time with their children. According to one study, the less time parents spent with their children, the more they spent to buy them items like videos and toys

(Schembari, 1999). In either case, shopping becomes a proxy. But the feelings of satisfaction are fleeting—as Krueger writes, "it's like treating appendicitis with morphine. It doesn't resolve the conflict" (quoted in Rozhon, 1998). To assist his prospective patients at recognizing the symptoms of shopping disorder, Dr. Krueger offers a self-help quiz:

- Do you go shopping to escape feeling bored, empty, angry, or scared?
- Do you use shopping or spending in a way that creates conflicts for you, or between you and others?
- Do you buy things with your credit cards that you wouldn't buy if you had the cash?
- When you shop or make a purchase, does your mood change—do you feel euphoric or anxious?

A shopper answering yes to any of these questions, he writes, is likely to be using shopping as a way to regulate their self-esteem. Readers may recognize several of these symptoms in the way we all shop sometimes. The certainly give us pause to consider whether American society does not collectively suffer from dysfunctional shopping disorder.

Meanwhile, debts have been mounting for those who cannot afford it. Overall, credit card debt as a percentage of household disposable income has risen 60 percent since 1989. Total household debt grew from 56 percent of disposable personal income in 1983 to 81 percent by the beginning of 1995. Commercial banks sent out 2.7 billion preapproved credit card solicitations in 1995—an average of seventeen to every American between ages eighteen and sixty-four (Frank, 1999). A recent study conducted by the Survey Research Unit of the Ohio State University College of Social and Behavioral Sciences found, not surprisingly, that carrying credit card debt was a significant source of stresses and worries. Credit card debt, unlike debt acquired from the purchase of homes and cars, can be uniquely stressful for two reasons: first, because almost all credit card debt is unsecured debt, meaning that there is no collateral secured on the debt. This may lead to more aggressive collection tactics by banks when lenders default on payments. Second, credit card debt is considered nonnormative compared with "normative" debts such as a home mortgage. While debt incurred from a home and car are deemed necessities in American society, credit card debt is often viewed as "excessive" debt taken on by those with prodigal habits, even if such debts in reality are those incurred by individuals who have suffered a recent job loss or health problems. In the Ohio study, the ratio of credit card debt to family income was an even stronger predictor of poor self-rated health than low personal income (Drentea and Lavrakas, 2000).

In turn, credit card debt has been blamed for the increase in bankruptcy cases in the United States (Cocheo, 1997). Personal bankruptcy filings rose throughout the 1990s. Nationwide, 29,000 personal bankruptcy filings are made each week. More spending means less saving. By all accounts, the nation is experiencing a savings crisis. One-third of Americans have no savings at all, and the next third have less than $3,000 in savings. Although baby boomers have contributed to the explosion of investment in securities, only two in five of them will have enough savings to maintain their living standard when they begin to retire in 2011 (Coverdell and Torricelli, 1999). The U.S. ranks last among the five largest OECD countries in net savings as a percentage of net national income (Figure 4.4).

FIGURE 4.4

NET SAVINGS AS A PERCENTAGE
OF NATIONAL INCOME
IN FIVE OECD COUNTRIES

(FROM FRANK, 1999)

	1970s	1980s	1990–92
Japan	25.6	20.9	23.0
Germany	15.1	11.2	12.4
France	17.1	9.0	8.7
Italy	16.4	11.2	7.6
U.S.A.	9.1	5.2	2.5
All OECD	13.8	9.7	8.7

Net savings in Japan were three times higher than in the United States in the 1970s; by 1990–92, they were more than nine times as high. In 1998, American's personal savings rate fell to a post–World War II low of 0.5 percent of disposable income. We spent 99.5 percent of our after-tax income (Samuelson, 1999). By the summer of 1999, personal spending was rising at twice the pace of incomes. The savings rate in July 2000 fell to minus 0.2 percent, the lowest level since government records started in 1959 (*The New York Times,* August 29, 2000, p. C2).

Consumer spending finally slowed down in response to the falling stock market and rising layoffs of 2001. For the first time since 1992, the Federal Reserve announced that outstanding consumer credit remained stable, at around $1.59 trillion, during the quarter from May to August, 2001 (Leonhardt and Atlas, 2001). Paradoxically, as American consumers cut back on their personal spending and begin to save for a rainy day, they threaten to choke off the engine that drove the recent economic boom. As everyone is reminded now, especially since the September 11 terrorist attacks, it is our patriotic duty to borrow and spend.

CONSUMER DEBT AND THE CHARITY CRUNCH

The ultimate example of how consumer dissaving has hurt our fellow Americans can be found in the decline of charitable gift-giving. Even as the incomes of the better-off Americans soared in the recent economic boom, charities across the nation reported that both individuals and companies were donating less to organizations that support the homeless and the hungry (Kilborn, 1999). Apparently, being in debt leaves the average American family with less to give to those in need. To be sure, overall gifts to charity surged to record levels, to $203 billion in 2000, more than double the amount a decade earlier, when the $100 billion threshold was first topped (Lewin, 2001). But at the same time, the growth in charitable giving failed to match the growth in the economy, or in personal incomes. According to a spokesman from the White House Office of Faith-Based and Community Initiatives: "If people at the [twentieth] century's end gave the way their parents did in the 1950s, we would have an extra $20 billion annually in good works" (quoted in Lewin, 2001). Similarly, a report by a San Francisco–based philanthropic research organization, the New Tithing Group, estimated that Americans with gross incomes of $1 million or more could have afforded to give ten times more than their actual donations.

About 90 percent of charitable giving goes to religious organizations (some of which operate services to the poor), as well as to other organizations that cater mostly to the rich, such as the opera, ballet, museums, and universities. Leaders of charitable organizations have been complaining that donors seem more willing these days to give for buildings and endowments than for services to the poor.

No one keeps track of contributions to programs targeted to the poor. But Giving USA estimates that contributions for human services, including most forms of traditional charity, actually fell from 13.9 percent in 1970 to 9.2 percent of all giving by 1998. Similarly, the Independent Sector, a coalition of philanthropic organizations, reported that households donated just 2.1 percent of their incomes in 1998, compared with 2.5 percent a decade ago, and that the number of those making any contributions fell to 70.1 percent from 75.1 percent in 1989 (Kilborn, 1999).

Even before the end of the most recent economic boom in America, the need for food at soup kitchens and food pantries had been growing bigger, not smaller. As food stamp eligibility declined following the passage of the 1996 Welfare Reform Act, the trend was matched by growing queues at community food banks. In Arizona, between March 1994 and July 1998, as participation in the food-stamp program fell by more than 50 percent, there was a parallel 50 percent jump in meals distributed through the state's charity network (Revkin, 1999a). Even in communities that are relatively flush with donations, the assortment of foods often failed to match those that were most needed, such as cereals and pasta. The Neighbor to Neighbor food pantry in Greenwich, Connecticut, reportedly featured a "gourmet" section that included items such as goose liver pâté, lemon curd, and bamboo shoots (Revkin, 1999b). The sense of starvation amidst plenty was never so poignant.

Charity executives profess to be puzzled by why Americans do not seem willing to share more of their prosperity with the poor. Notwithstanding the outpouring of generosity demonstrated towards the families of the victims of the September 11 tragedy, Americans seem less attuned to the needs of the poor living just around the corner. In the words of Herman Ewing, president of the Urban League of Memphis:

> Prosperity, for all its appeal, can undermine the sharing and the bonds of neighbors and communities and gives people a lot to protect. . . . The result of prosperity is isolation, arrogance, and in-your-face. This among people who were once interdependent in terms of basic survival needs. The idea that you're looking out for me for food and I'm looking out for you for this or that is all by the boards (Kilborn, 1999).

CHAPTER FIVE

INEQUALITY—
THE PRIVATE AND
PUBLIC PRICE
WE PAY

IS INEQUALITY GOOD FOR PRODUCTIVITY?

American culture places a high value on competition. We tolerate inequalities because it spurs individuals to try their best. The greater the extent of inequality, so the argument goes, the greater the incentive to strive harder. Economists are fond of pointing out that player performance tends to be higher in professional golf tournaments, where the spread in the size of prize money is wider (Ehrenberg and Bognanno, 1990). Similarly, the performance of professional auto racers have been found to be related not just to the size of the prize money, but also to the degree of spread between finishing-place prizes (Becker and Huselid, 1992). According to this view, life is one big tournament, in which we are players vying for the top prizes.

A review of American public opinion data over fifty years concluded: "Surveys since the 1930s have shown that the explicit idea of income redistribution elicits very limited enthusiasm among the American public. . . . Redistributive fervor was not much apparent even in [the] depression era. Most Americans are content with the distributional effects of private markets" (Lipset, 1997). American citizens have a greater tendency than others to take a benign view of income differences, as judged by cross-national reactions to the statement that "Large income differences are needed for the country's prosperity" (Lipset, 1997, p. 73). Inequality is thus viewed as the engine of growth.

One of the most famous arguments made on behalf of the positive benefits of inequality was laid down by two sociologists, Kingsley Davis and Wilbert E. Moore. In their seminal 1945 article, Davis and Moore set forth the following sequential propositions:

(1) Certain positions in society are functionally more important than others, and require special skills for their performance.

(2) Only a limited number of individuals in any society have the talents that can be trained into the skills required for those positions.

(3) The conversion of talents into skills involves a period of training during which sacrifices of one kind or another must be made by those undergoing the training.

(4) In order to induce the talented persons to undergo these sacrifices, their future positions must carry an inducement value in the form of privileged and disproportionate access to the scarce and desired rewards that society has to offer, e.g., pay, prestige, respect.

(5) Therefore, inequality among different social strata in the amounts of scarce and desired goods is both positively functional, desirable, and inevitable in any society.

No doubt about it—these are a set of seemingly hard-to-refute arguments that have been countlessly rehearsed by defenders of the free market ever since. But if inequality is positively functional in the sense that Davis and Moore described, what is the actual evidence that it leads to desirable economic outcomes? Back in Chapter 3, we referred to the international evidence that suggested that income inequality is linked to higher risks of premature death. But what if inequality is *good* for society in other respects, such as increased productivity and economic growth? Might improvements in economic performance offset any undesirable effects on population health? Might Americans be willing to make such trade-offs? After all, people are frequently willing to trade off their health status for improvements in their standard of living (as, for example, when workers take on risky jobs for more "hazard pay"). What, then, does the research tell us about economic inequality as an incentive for better productivity and performance? To answer that question, let us turn to America's favorite pastime: major-league baseball.

It certainly takes a phenomenal amount of talent and effort to make it to the major leagues. Few of us would begrudge the high salaries earned by our top professional baseball players whose careers reflect an extraordinary winnowing process beginning with successes in T-ball and Little League, then moving on to the Babe Ruth League, competitive high school teams, and finally on to the minor leagues. Even for the select few who make it to the minor leagues, only a fraction of them end up being picked for the major-league rosters, and among those, even fewer eventually land a starting berth. What could be a better incentive in this highly competitive market than to offer megasalaries for those who make it to the top?

The fact, however, is that multimillion-dollar salaries are a comparatively recent phenomenon in major-league baseball. For most of their history, major professional sports leagues cooperated under regulations that forbade franchise owners from bidding for each other's star players. Major league baseball was no exception—at least until the mid-1970s when it became the first professional sport to abandon its reserve clause after a series of legal challenges. Since then, as we all know, major-league player salaries have sky-rocketed (Figure 5.1).

The average player's salary was more than 3,700 percent greater in 1993 than it was in 1976. It is now more than fifty times the average per capita income in the United States, up from only eight times in 1976 (Frank and Cook, 1995). Inequality within major-league teams keeps growing, just like the rest of America. According to *USA Today*'s year 2000 annual salary survey, just 14 percent of the players accounted for more than half the player payroll for the thirty major-league clubs on opening day (www.usatoday.com/sports/baseball/salary). In 2000, the L.A. Dodgers signed on the pitcher Kevin Brown for a record $15.7 million, nearly $5.8 million more than the next highest paid player on the team, Gary Sheffield. Presumably, the management of the Dodgers hoped that by signing on Brown, they would induce the pitcher to strive harder and to lift his team's performance. What is the evidence that incentive pay of this magnitude produces higher performance?

To test this hypothesis, Matt Bloom, assistant professor of

FIGURE 5.1

TRENDS IN AVERAGE MAJOR-LEAGUE
BASEBALL SALARIES 1976–2000

Average Salary ($ millions)

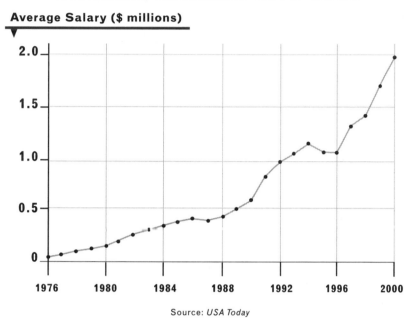

Source: *USA Today*

management at the University of Notre Dame (and a baseball
fan) carried out an analysis of 1,644 baseball players on twenty-
nine teams over the period 1985 through 1993. Every year, *USA
Today* publishes the salaries of all the major-league baseball players. For each team, Bloom calculated the extent of dispersion in
players' salaries. If Moore and Davis are right, then the greater
the extent of inequality in salaries, the higher the amount of effort that managers ought to be able to coax out of their players,
and consequently the better the team performance.

Bloom measured individual player performance using several well-established indicators: for hitters, the adjusted batting

runs, fielding runs, and total player rating; and for pitchers, the adjusted earned run average, pitching runs, and total pitcher rating. As anyone who follows baseball statistics knows, these numbers are quite rigorously calculated. For example, the adjusted batting runs is calculated by the formula: $(0.47 \times \text{singles}) + (0.78 \times \text{doubles}) + (1.09 \times \text{triples}) + (1.40 \times \text{home runs}) + (0.33 \times \text{bases on balls} + \text{number of times hit as a batsman}) - (0.25 \times (\text{at bats} - \text{hits})) - (0.5 \times \text{outs on base})$. And so on.

To gauge team (as opposed to individual) performance, he used the winning percentage (wins per game played), fan attendance, and the team's finishing position (number of games behind the division leader at the end of the season). Contrary to Davis and Moore's predictions, the wider the pay dispersion in any given team, the worse was the performance of individual players. Unequal pay distribution had significantly negative effects on player performance, over and above the effects of base pay, past performance, age, and experience. More tellingly, wider pay differentials translated into worse *team* performance. More unequal teams won fewer games, *and* they did worse financially in terms of fan attendance. For every 1.6 percent increase in the measure of pay dispersion, the team's winning percentage went down by 26 percent, and the attendance ratio (total home attendance divided by the stadium capacity times the number of home games) went down by a whopping 41 percent. Evidently, something is seriously awry with Moore and Davis's predictions.

What could account for Bloom's findings? Two possible explanations come to mind. One is that far from spurring individuals to do their best, wider pay gaps may instill feelings of unfairness ("Is he *really* worth $3.5 million more than me?"), promote dissatisfaction and resentment, and ultimately diminish individual (and hence team) performance. Such disincentives may be felt especially by players who are lower down on the pay scale (indeed, Bloom found this to be the case).

A second explanation for Bloom's findings is that wider pay dispersion creates disincentives against cooperation, especially in a game that frequently relies on teamwork (such as turning double plays or defending against bunts). In a world in which each individual is looking out for themselves, players will tend to concentrate on improving their own performance to the exclusion of team goals, since their own performance is what matters for moving up the pay scale. Concentrating on trying to hit more home runs or improving one's own hitting average are not necessarily the tactics that lift team performance—as opposed to, say, practicing great defense. Outside of major-league baseball, individuals may even engage in dysfunctional behaviors such as sabotaging the work of fellow employees in an effort to garner more of the organization's compensation resources. In sum, inequalities in compensation may lead to less cooperation, less team-oriented behavior, lower common goal orientation, and active erosion of social cohesion.

Although the example of major-league baseball may strike some readers as somewhat fanciful, Bloom's research has obvious implications for a much wider segment of the labor market. In manufacturing firms, wider pay dispersion has been found to result in lower product quality (Cowherd and Levine, 1992). In American manufacturing firms, the average compensation of a CEO can be up to 150 times that of the average worker, much higher than the salaries of their counterparts in Japan or Germany. Whereas American CEOs routinely lay off thousands of workers during economic downturns (and reward themselves in the process for "increasing efficiency"), their Japanese counterparts have been known to take voluntary pay cuts to preserve jobs. One may wonder how these different practices translate in terms of the quality of, say, American and Japanese automobiles. When Daimler-Benz announced in May 1998 that it would acquire the Chrysler Corporation, the CEO of Daimler was earning much less than his counterpart at Chrysler, a much smaller company. Soon after the acquisition of Chrysler by Daimler, the German company was forced to announce a change in its system of executive compensation (Bryant, 1999). Research informs us that a foreseeable consequence of creating a more cutthroat managerial environment is reduced employee commitment stemming from more antagonistic social relations, and more workforce instability in the form of lower managerial tenure and higher turnover (Bloom, 2000). Thus, while wider pay hierarchies may cultivate star performers, they come at a cost of reduced workplace stability and cohesion.

All of this is not to suggest that wide pay differentials are universally undesirable. They may be quite appropriate in organizations that have low demands for cooperation, such as stock brokerages or law firms. But they are quite likely to be detrimental in organizations that require any significant degree of cooperation, such as manufacturing teams, firefighting squads, hotel customer-service staffs, and many others (Bloom, 1999). The truth about economic inequality is much more complex than suggested by Davis and Moore.

WINNER-TAKE-ALL MARKETS

Now that we have seen that inequality can be quite dysfunctional in terms of an organization's performance, we turn to the costs of inequality for the economy as a whole. The pay structure of major-league baseball follows a pattern of what Robert Frank and Philip Cook dubbed "winner-take-all" markets (Frank and Cook, 1995). These markets are the logical consequence of the kind of arguments advanced by Davis and Moore: In order to attract the top talent into the top positions, we need to pay them more—a lot more. Whereas we have grown quite accustomed to seeing winner-take-all markets in professional sports and Hollywood movie stars' paychecks, Frank and Cook contend that they have become much more widespread across the rest of American society, contributing to widening income disparities. Thus, we see features of winner-take-all markets in banking, law firms, consulting, journalism, medicine, publishing, corporate management, and even academic institutions.

As Frank and Cook concede, for any nation to prosper in the face of growing international competition, it must somehow allocate its most talented citizens to its most important jobs (the Davis and Moore argument, again). This means:

> It must steer its best executives to the enterprises that add greatest value, its most creative scientists to the most pressing technical problems, its ablest public servants to the most important cabinet positions. If the economic collapse of the communist countries can be traced to any single factor, it is their dismal performance in these critical assignment tasks. The critics of communism were right all along. The allocation of talent by central bureaucracies is a recipe for economic disaster (Frank and Cook, p. 7).

But before we give ourselves a pat on our backs for winning the Cold War, the same economists hasten to point out two important senses in which winner-take-all markets can also be socially wasteful. First, such markets, in their extreme form, can lead to the paradoxical *misallocation* of talent. The problem arises because if every contestant in a winner-take-all market chooses to compete for the finite number of top positions, too few will end up seeking productive careers in more mundane (but socially necessary) markets. In other words, "our national income would be higher if some students abandon their ambitions to become multimillionaire plaintiffs' attorneys in favor of the more modest but more predictable paychecks of electrical engineers." A second sense in which winner-take-all markets can be wasteful is when contestants end up engaging in a veritable arms race of investment and consumption spending whilst clawing their way to the top.

Take the example of spending on getting higher education credentials from elite academic organizations. By now, many parents understand that the top positions in winner-take-all markets are all but closed to those who do not have degrees from the most prestigious academic institutions, preferably an Ivy League school. Worrying about building a résumé that will get their offspring admitted into one of these top universities has intensified the pressure among middle-class parents to engage in what *Newsweek* recently termed "scheduled hyperactivity." Take a typical week in the life of the Lee family in Minneapolis, as profiled in that magazine:

> The three oldest kids—Anna, 12, Nathan, 9, and Kristian, 7—play one sport or another practically all year round. . . . Anna's the complete jock, participating in soccer, volleyball, basketball and softball. Nathan and Kristian do it all except volleyball. In the summer, add on tennis and swim lessons.

All of which means that Dad, Darwin, a teacher, and Mom, JoΛnn, a nurse, spend an incredible amount of time making sure everyone gets where he needs to be. Family dinners? Forget about it. "I wish we had more downtime," says Darwin, somewhat wistfully. "It seems like Anna is running off almost every night. . . . I miss seeing her. I miss talking to her" (*Newsweek,* July 17, 2000, p. 49).

In the view of one expert quoted in the same article, if parents and kids don't make time for each other, emotional ties will wither and die: "We now have a more competitive society, a more consumerist society, and these forces influence families. Raising kids becomes like product development. It's competitive parenting, all well intentioned, to develop the kid in every possible way."

We shall return to the malaise of loosening family and community bonds in a later chapter, and merely note for the moment that if every middle-class family in America decided to do as the Lee family in Minneapolis do, everyone would end up being more stressed but in exactly the same relative position that they were in before with respect to glittering résumés.

From the supply side, also, winner-take-all markets have resulted in an escalation of defensive spending. Responding to the successes of our top academic institutions, less prestigious universities across the country have started to mimic the strategy of bidding for star faculty and top administrators. Top administrators' salaries have sky-rocketed on the basis of their ability to raise funds and increase school enrollment. These costs, in turn, get passed on to parents in the form of escalating tuition fees. Undergraduate tuition at Ivy League schools (excluding room, board, and living expenses) was less than $3,000 per year back in the seventies; now it is up to $30,000 and rising. Yet if the number of places at elite institutions remains unchanged, everyone is spending more to end up in exactly the same position.

How did we end up in this mess in the first place? The arms race on educational spending applies not only to our elite institutions but also to higher education in general. Considered in isolation, an individual's spending on a higher education degree should improve his or her chances of getting a desirable job. Acting alone, each individual seeks to make the best of his or her position. But there is also a "pollution" element in an individual's expenditure on education. That is because the value of spending on a given level of education as a means of access to the most sought-after jobs will decline as more people attain the same level of education. As the economist Fred Hirsch pointed out: "The value to me of my education depends not only on how much I have but also on how much the man ahead of me in the job line has" (Hirsch, 1976; p. 3). The satisfaction of an individual's preference for higher educational status in itself alters the situation for *others* seeking to satisfy similar wants. A round of transactions to act out personal wants of this kind therefore leaves each individual in exactly the same position as before, since there are only a limited number of the most desirable jobs. What each of us can achieve in isolation, all cannot.

Faced with an increase in the number of qualified applicants, employers respond by allocating the most attractive positions through increased screening. In practice, this means the escalation of education credentials: the job formerly open to college graduates now demands a master's degree, or a degree from an elite university. This credentialing process, in turn, forces ever more Americans to engage in what Hirsch called "defensive" spending. Individuals who decline to join the educational upgrading will suffer a devaluation of their credentials in terms of their job access. Then, "education becomes a good investment, not because it would raise an individual's income above what it would have been if no one had increased their education, but because it raises their income above what it would be if others acquire an education and they do not" (Thurow and Lucas, 1972). The vicious circle is closed when an expansion in the supply of qualified applicants further raises the threshold of necessary credentials. An inflation of educational credentials of this kind involves social waste in two dimensions: first, because of the disappointed expectations of individuals, and from the frustration they feel in having to settle for a job in which they cannot make full use of their acquired skills; and secondly, because competition of this sort absorbs real resources that could have been better expended elsewhere.

In the 1980s, one in five college graduates in America ended up in jobs that the Bureau of Labor Statistics defines as not requiring a college degree: sales clerks, typists, file clerks, and laborers. This figure compares with the one in ten college graduates who were overqualified for their jobs in the late 1960s. Based on the ongoing glut of college enrollments, Labor Department economists have predicted that by the year 2005, nearly 30 percent of the nation's college graduates will be working as file clerks, assembly workers, or some other occupation that does not require higher education (Newman, 1993).

Higher education has often been linked in the public's eye with the societal benefits it confers. Such benefits are based on the assumption that educated people make better citizens—that they are more productive, and that they enhance the productivity of those with whom they work. Moreover, such benefits are not all captured in the higher earnings of educated individuals.

On the other hand, the deadweight losses imposed by positional spending on education will necessarily diminish the value of such external benefits. Their presence means that the increase in *personal* productivity as measured by market earnings is not matched by an increase in *social* productivity:

> Education adds to personal earnings, but not commensu- rably to social product. . . . To the extent that education con- veys information about the . . . *relative* capacity of the individual who has undergone it, more education for all leaves everyone in the same place.

> [I]t is a case of everyone in the crowd standing on tiptoe and no one getting a better view. Yet at the start of the process some individuals gain a better view by standing on tiptoe, and others are forced to follow if they are to keep their position. If all do follow . . . everyone expends more resources and ends up with the same position (Hirsch, 1976; p. 49).

Of course, we are here *not* advocating that Americans should drop out of higher education—many valuable things can still be learned in our colleges and universities that doubtless enrich our personal lives as well as our shared national culture. Nor are we talking about the egregious inequalities that persist in the provi- sion of *basic* education across communities of the United States, as poignantly documented by writers like Jonathan Kozol (1991). We are simply pointing out, as James K. Galbraith (1998) has done, that higher educational investment is often touted for the wrong reason. Social reformers on both sides of the political spectrum are fond of advocating more investment in higher education as a remedy for stagnant wages and the rising disparities in income that we described in Chapter 1. Investing in higher education will supposedly help poor Americans overcome the "skill bias" in technological change, which has been blamed as the main culprit behind the growing disparities in pay.

But as Galbraith argues, investing in higher education is not the remedy for stagnant wages and growing inequalities:

> Will the provision of resources [for higher education], if it can be achieved, matter much for the *average* level of American economic performance? . . . Can we get to a higher sustained rate of economic growth, and a material improvement in national living standards, merely by pumping up the resources we devote to education? *That* question turns on whether there is a shortage of skilled labor in the United States, a shortage not being met by our colleges and universities. Despite all the ruminations about "skill bias" in the patterns of technological change, there is no such shortage. To the contrary, our economy is full of highly educated and skilled people. *It remains short of jobs for those people,* as every college counselor and every coordinator of a training program knows (Galbraith, 1998; p. 208, emphasis added).

Nor for that matter is there anything wrong with a job flipping hamburgers or bagging groceries. The problem in the United States is not that we have too many low-skilled "bad" jobs, but that we have a shortage of more skilled "good" jobs for entry-level workers to graduate into (Freeman, 1997). This point, overlooked by those who advocate "educational investment," was obvious even to an eleven-year-old boy interviewed by Jay MacLeod in his study of kids from Clarendon Heights, a low-income housing project in a northeastern city. As the boy tells the interviewer, "I ain't going to college. Who wants to go to college? I'd just end up gettin' a shitty job anyway" (MacLeod, 1987). Such an opinion offends our sensibilities and contradicts the American achievement ideology, which maintains that any child can grow up to become Andrew Carnegie. Yet what the ideology conveniently ignores is what happened to Carnegie's classmates, the bulk of whom failed to rise above their parents' stations. Given the scarcity of desirable jobs and the dynamics of positional competition, the mantra of "educational investment" has the hollow ring of supply-side economics.

THE DYSFUNCTIONS OF INEQUALITY—
A REBUTTAL TO DAVIS AND MOORE

Inequality is not necessarily functional (as in coaxing higher productivity out of individuals), nor always socially desirable (as in maximizing the efficiency of allocating society's scarce resources). It looks like Davis and Moore were wrong on both counts. There is no necessary trade-off between equity and efficiency, at least within the range of income distribution under which we currently operate. On the other hand, we have identified several dysfunctional aspects of inequality, which were best summarized in a famous rebuttal to Davis and Moore by the sociologist Melvin Tumin (1953):

(1) Social inequalities function to limit the possibility of discovery of the full range of talent available in a society. This results from the unequal access to opportunities, especially education and training.

(2) Social inequalities function to provide the elite in a society with the political power necessary to procure acceptance and dominance of an ideology that rationalizes the status quo as "logical," "natural," and "morally right."

(3) To the extent that inequalities in social rewards cannot be made fully acceptable to the less privileged in society, social inequalities function to encourage hostility, suspicion, and distrust among the various segments of society and thus to limit the possibilities of extensive social integration.

(4) To the extent that participation depends on the sense of significant membership in the society, social inequalities cause social exclusion and function to distribute the motivation to participate unequally in a population.

INEQUALITY AND DEATH REVISITED

Now that we have established that the degree of inequality in America is neither functional nor socially desirable, we are ready to revisit the subject of health and well-being. Back in Chapter 3, we talked about the cross-country evidence that income inequality may be associated with lower health achievement. A skeptic might point out that this evidence simply reflects historical, cultural, and other differences between countries that determine their overall health achievement. However, when we examine the relationship between income inequality and health *within* a single country like the United States, exactly the same pattern is revealed. A series of studies has been published in recent years that demonstrate higher rates of mortality and lower levels of well-being among states with wider dispersion of household incomes.

In two American studies published simultaneously in 1996, George Kaplan and colleagues from the University of Michigan, and our own team at the Harvard School of Public Health, tested the relationship between income inequality and variations in premature death rates across the fifty U.S. states. Kaplan and colleagues used as their measure of income distribution the share of total income earned by the bottom 50 percent of households in each state. If incomes were perfectly equally shared, the bottom half of households should account for exactly half of the total income earned by all of the households in each state (we are not claiming this to be a desirable goal—it is just a convenient benchmark). In reality, the proportion of total income earned by the bottom half of households ranged from a minimum of 17.5 percent (in Louisiana, the most unequal) to a high of 23.6 percent (New Hampshire, the most egalitarian). A highly significant correlation ($r = -0.62$) was found between this measure of inequality and premature death rates, which was present in both men and women, and in white Americans as well as African-Americans. The other study, by Kennedy, Kawachi, and Prothrow-Stith (1996), examined two measures of income distribution: the Gini coefficient and the Robin Hood Index. The Gini index is perhaps the most widely used measure of income distribution, and theoretically ranges from 0.0 (perfect equality) to 1.0 (perfect inequality). The Robin Hood Index can be interpreted as the proportion of aggregate income that must be redistributed from rich to poor households in order to attain perfect equality of incomes across households. Like the study by Kaplan and colleagues, both measures were strikingly correlated with death rates (Figure 5.2).

FIGURE 5.2

THE RELATIONSHIP OF INCOME INEQUALITY
TO MORTALITY RATES ACROSS THE U.S.

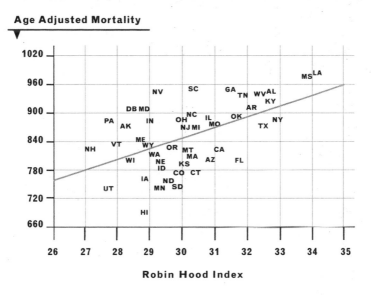

Source: Kaplan, et al.

Even after taking account of state differences in poverty rates and median household income, each 1 percent increase in the Robin Hood Index was associated with an excess death rate of about 22 deaths per 100,000 population. Greater inequality in the distribution of income was associated with not just higher rates of overall mortality, but also rates of premature death from heart attack, cancer, murder, and infant mortality. Income inequality and poverty rates could together explain about one quarter of the variation across the states in overall mortality rates, as well as just over half of the variation in murder rates.

More recently, John Lynch and colleagues (1998) have extended the investigation of income inequality and death rates down to the level of metropolitan areas within the United States. The researchers calculated income inequality indices for 282 U.S. metropolitan areas, ranging in population size from 56,735 for Enid, Oklahoma, to 18,087,251 for New York. They found that metropolitan areas with high income inequality and low per capita income had an excess death rate of about 140 deaths per 100,000 compared with that of areas with low inequality and high per capita income. This mortality difference was estimated by the authors to be comparable in size to eliminating all deaths from lung cancer, diabetes, motor vehicle crashes, AIDS, suicide, and homicide in this country. Even a modest reduction in inequality could thus have an important impact on public health.

What is the reason that income inequality should be linked to mortality rates in this way? Part of the answer lies in the shape of the relationship between income and mortality rates. As we observed back in Chapter 3, one of the universally observed characteristics of the relationship linking income to health status is that it is *curved*. The slope is quite steep near the bottom of the income distribution (for example, see Figure 3.4). At very low levels of income, the risk of death drops quite quickly with each additional increment in earnings (or conversely, average life expectancy rises quite quickly with each additional dollar of GDP—see Figure 3.1). Having an extra dollar can make an important difference to the health of the poor. However, as more and more income is earned, the *slope* of the curve starts to level off—in other words, there are diminishing returns to additional income. Even though the gradient linking income to mortality extends well into what we would consider the "middle-class" range of household income, the fact remains that making an extra few thousand dollars is going to make less of a difference to the life expectancy of a Forbes 400 executive than to a welfare mother. Now, an important consequence of what we have just said is that the *distribution* of income must influence the average life expectancy of a society. The tendency for greater dispersion of income to be associated with lower average life expectancy can be illustrated by considering a hypothetical society consisting of just two individuals—a rich one with income x_4, and a poor one with income x_1. The average income is therefore x (Figure 5.3).

In this society, income is steeply related to life expectancy on the left-hand side of x, but the curve levels off toward the right. Reading off this chart, the mean life expectancy in this society would be y_1 (the average between the rich and poor individual). Now let's imagine what would happen if a new tax law was in-

FIGURE 5.3

THE CONCAVE RELATIONSHIP BETWEEN INCOME AND LIFE EXPECTANCY

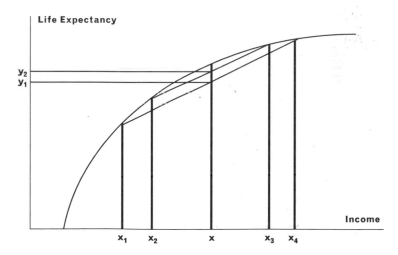

troduced, such that a certain amount of money (the amount x_4 minus x_3) was transferred from the affluent individual to raise the income of the poor individual (from x_1 to x_2). We now see that the average life expectancy in this hypothetical society has risen to y_2. In other words, a more egalitarian distribution of income resulted in an increase in average life expectancy, even though the *average* level of income remained same. By extending this argument, we might expect that two societies with the same average income but different distributions of income would vary in their level of health achievement, with the more egalitarian society exhibiting higher life expectancy. There is no legerdemain involved in this—the prediction is simply a consequence of the concave relation between income and life expectancy. In other words, an increase in life expectancy among the poor as a result of redistributing income more than offsets any health loss experienced by the affluent.

There are other important mechanisms by which income inequality lowers the health achievement of society that involve distortions in political participation and spending on social goods, which we shall turn to in a later chapter. For the moment, an important question is who ends up paying more for the cost of inequality—the poor or the rich? This is a different question from the scenario we have just been considering. In theory, it is possible that *both* the poor and rich will experience worse health outcomes as a result of living in a society with more unequal distribution of income. For instance, if there is more violent crime in an unequal society, the rich who live there might be more likely to become victims of homicide than their counterparts who live in more egalitarian, less violent societies. Although several studies have begun to address this question (Lochner, et al., 2001; Kahn, et al., 2000), the jury is still out in terms of a definitive answer. For example, Kimberly Lochner and colleagues (2001) followed up nearly 547,000 individuals in the U.S. National Health Interview Survey, and found that living in high inequality states was associated with increased death rates for the poor (those with incomes below the federal poverty threshold) as well as the near-poor (those with incomes up to double the poverty line), but not the non-poor. Using a different survey (the National Maternal Infant Health Survey) and a different health outcome (self-assessed health), Robert Kahn and colleagues found also that high inequality states most adversely affected the mental health of poor people. However, near the top of the income distribution, Kahn and colleagues found that inequality may actually *benefit* the rich, i.e., the affluent fare somewhat better as a result of taking up residence in a state where the gap between them and the rest of society is bigger. As other data become available, this question is sure to be revisited.

CHAPTER SIX

STEPPING ON THE HEDONIC TREADMILL

We pay twice over for the costs of maintaining a high degree of inequality—once as individuals, and again as a society. In the private domain, the surge in income inequality during the past twenty years has translated into individuals working longer hours and sending more family members to work—just to keep up with living standards in the face of stagnant and declining wages. Meanwhile, consumer society promises the attainment of happiness but ultimately fails to deliver. The pursuit of happiness is the proverbial carrot dangling on the end of the stick. We leap on the hedonic treadmill, only to discover that our insatiable wants remain unsatisfied, while our health suffers. More time at work has meant less time for leisure and less time spent with families and friends, reduced parental investment in children, and generally less of the types of consumption that really make a difference to our well-being. Striving harder has also led to frustration, especially for those who have little hope of achieving their dreams. The road to the American Dream is strewn with the unhappy lives of broken families, of lonely and overworked people who spend their free time in front of their television sets, being bombarded by commercials that advertise luxury automobiles, anniversary diamonds, vacation cruises, and other accessories of material success.

From the societal perspective, striving to catch up to an ever-rising standard of living has spawned a whole host of undesirable spill-over effects. More time at work has led to the withdrawal of citizens from all sorts of community participation. The greater the disparities in income distribution, the greater the erosion of social capital (Kawachi and Kennedy, 1997). In the relentless pursuit of lifestyles set by the rich, more and more Americans are living beyond their means and saving less. Living paycheck to paycheck has caused Americans to become less and less supportive of investments in public infrastructure financed through income taxation. Conspicuous consumption has crowded out so-called inconspicuous consumption—public spending on better roads, better schools, and improved neighborhoods—to the detriment of all (Frank, 1999). As for those near the bottom of the economic heap, consumer society has led to frustration (expressed in outbreaks of violence) or attempts to attain the desirable standard of living through any means possible, including the resort to a life of crime (Venkatesh, 1997). Nationwide, we incarcerate 1.8 million offenders, up from the figure of 330,000 in 1972 (Butterfield, 1999). Every twenty seconds, someone in America is arrested for a drug violation. Every week on average, a new jail or prison is built to lock up more people in the world's largest penal system (Egan, 1999). The state of California alone spends nearly $4 billion a year to operate the nation's largest prison system,

more than the gross national product of countries like Cambo-
dia ($3.2 billion), Haiti ($2.9 billion), and Namibia ($3.4 billion).
California added twenty-one prisons since 1984, and only one
university campus during the same period. Spending on prisons
grew 60 percent over the last decade, while pay for prison
guards more than doubled. A prison guard in that state now
makes about $51,000 a year, compared with $41,000 for a first-
year professor in one of California's state universities.

Meanwhile, to assuage their fear of crime, some 4 million
Americans now live in gated communities. Total American
spending on private security products and services topped $57
billion in 1996. New York City now spends $60,000 per year to
keep an adult incarcerated, and $70,000 for each juvenile—
more than ten times the amount the city spends per pupil in
public schools (Frank, 1999, p. 264).

Aside from crime, the wider the gulf between the haves and
have-nots, the more intense are the pressures caused by relative
deprivation, and the more extreme the manifestations of consumer society. The quest for bigger homes—McMansions—
has forced massive expansion of housing development into
rural areas, contributing to environmental degradation, hope-
lessly snarled traffic, and the instant creation of communities of
alienated residents. All of the undesirable spillover effects of
competitive striving described above are more prevalent in a society that exhibits greater disparities in wealth and incomes. We
now turn to a closer examination of these ills.

WORKING HARDER, FEELING WORSE

Part of the surge in income inequality during the 1980s and
1990s has been blamed on an increase in the "skill premium" in

American society, defined as the pay differential among workers with different levels of skill. Although the skill premium indeed widened during those decades, it hardly did so because the top earners pulled away from the rest of the pack. In fact, between 1979 and 1995, the real earnings of male college graduates remained essentially stagnant, increasing by just 1 percent. Meanwhile the earnings of both high school graduates and men with less than high school education declined, by 17 percent and 27 percent, respectively. The only group who experienced a gain in real earnings during the same period were female college graduates (by 20 percent), which probably represents the movement of women into management, law, medicine, and similar high-paying occupations. The wages of female high school graduates and those with less than high school education dropped by 4 percent and 11 percent, respectively (Freeman, 1997).

Some have argued that the statistics on stagnating wages fail to take account of benefits provided by employers, like pensions, health insurance, and other fringe benefits (Cox and Alm, 1999). It is true that college graduates are more than twice as likely to receive employer-funded benefits than workers with less than high school education, so that the living standards of the most skilled workers may not have dropped off quite as much as the unskilled. But once again, a closer examination of trends in employer-provided benefits reveal that they also declined for all groups between 1979 and 1993. For college graduates, the probability that a worker was covered by an employer-funded pension or health insurance plan was 12 percent lower in 1993 than in 1979 if he was male, and 9 percent lower if she was female. (For the least skilled groups, the corresponding declines in coverage were 14 and 10 percent, respectively.)

American workers have responded to the reality of high earnings inequality, stagnant wages, and job insecurity by putting in longer hours at work. According to one calculation, production and nonsupervisory employees—who make up 80 percent of the American labor force—must now work an extra 245 hours, or 6-plus extra weeks per year, just to keep up with their 1973 standard of living (Schor, 1991). (Interestingly, some conservative views put the cart before the horse by arguing that higher taxes are forcing working people to put in longer hours!) In the past, the United States led the world in reductions of working time. It was among the first countries to establish the forty-hour week and to give paid vacation to ordinary workers. As recently as 1970, Americans worked fewer hours than Germans. But as inequality has risen over the past twenty years, and wages have stagnated, Americans have chosen more work over leisure. Compared with Europeans, employees in the United States in the mid-1990s worked two hundred to four hundred more hours during the year, a difference of five to ten full weeks. According to OECD estimates, Americans put in 1,952 hours in 1995, compared with 1,737 hours for the Canadians, 1,735 for the British, 1,631 hours for the French, 1,559 hours for Germans, and 1,544 hours for the Swedes. Americans now work more hours than the fabled workaholics of Japan, who logged in at 1,898 hours (Mishel, et al., 1999).

Any American who has traveled to Europe and tried to do some last-minute shopping before heading back home will discover that store hours over there are far more restricted than at home. If it happens to be a Sunday, the tourist is bound to be disappointed. Once again, we note the cultural connections between income disparities, longer work-hours, and a more intense consumer culture. It was only as recently as November

1996 that German laws were changed to permit retail stores to stay open on weekdays past 6:30 P.M. Stores there are still not allowed to stay open later than 8 P.M. on weekdays and 4 P.M. on Saturdays, while Sundays (as in much of the rest of Europe) remain entirely off-limits. Whereas retailers with a more American attitude might have approached this liberalization of laws as an opportunity to engage in open competition, German shopkeepers and merchants across the country banded together to develop cooperative rules about how long to stay open. In the five hundred-year-old village of Hofheim, near Frankfurt, shopkeepers decided that their stores would close no later than 7:30 P.M. on weekdays and 2 P.M. on Saturdays. Even so, many shopkeepers and store clerks were reported to be worried about getting home later for dinner and perhaps even having to give up the hallowed midday rest—the *Mittagspause*—that stretches between 12:30 and 2 P.M. (Andrews, 1996).

It might be pointed out that a major reason why American stores operate longer hours than German ones is that dual earner families are much more common here than in Europe. Thus Germans have tended to rely more on the traditional pattern of housewives doing the shopping on weekday mornings. As the number of German families with two working parents has climbed (up by one-third since the mid-1980s; now 46 percent of all households with children), the pressure for liberalizing store hours has predictably increased.

One major reason Americans work longer than Europeans is because they take less vacation—the average vacation days provided by American employers (about sixteen days per year), falls substantially below the statutory minimum holidays guaranteed in most European countries (between four and five weeks). In addition, 6 percent of Americans hold a second job; 18 percent of workers do job-related work at home; and overtime hours have risen substantially. The fact that international comparisons of GDP per capita do not take account of time worked means that American living standards are overstated compared with those in Europe. Americans have more material possessions than Europeans but less free time to enjoy them (Freeman, 1997).

Readers with Stakhanovite tendencies may question the relevance of vacations for health and well-being. After all, what could be the harm of being committed to one's job and contributing to the national output? In fact, epidemiological evidence suggests that not taking vacation is a risk factor for heart attack. The Framingham Heart Study is one of the nation's longest-running and most widely cited investigations of the causes of heart attack and cardiovascular diseases. The study was one of the first to convincingly demonstrate that cigarette smoking, high cholesterol, high blood pressure, and obesity are major risk factors for heart attack. According to twenty-year follow-up data from the same study, taking infrequent vacations is also a risk factor for developing heart attack (Eaker, et al., 1992). Compared with people who reported taking two or more vacations per year, those who took vacations only once every two to five years doubled their risk of heart attack. And those who took vacation only once every six or more years were at nearly eight times the risk of heart attack. The increased risk from taking infrequent vacations was found after controlling for other well-established risk factors for heart attack, including cigarette smoking, high blood pressure, serum cholesterol levels, diabetes, and obesity. Of note, individuals in the same study who reported high levels of psychological tension also tripled their risk of heart attack. It seems that taking a relaxing massage on board a cruise ship is good for the soul and your coronary arteries—provided you can afford to take the time off work.

THE TIME SQUEEZE

Americans are not only spending more hours at their jobs; at the same time, the demands of household labor have not diminished over time. When economist Juliet Schor (1991) examined long-term national trends in the annual hours Americans spent on both market and household work, she discovered that women worked on average 22 percent more hours in their paid jobs in 1987 than they did in 1969. To compensate, men did more housework in 1987 than they did in 1969, though still only roughly two-thirds the total hours that women put in (Figure 6.1). Combining both market and household hours of work, American women and men worked an extra month longer in 1987 than they did in 1969.

The growing pressure on working women to work the "double shift" has inevitably led to marital tensions and parental guilt over child-rearing, as documented by scholars like Arlie Hochschild (1989). Among several revealing interviews conducted by Hochschild in her groundbreaking study of working parents juggling the demands of paid work and housework, we meet Ann Myerson, a thirty-four-year-old vice president of a Silicon Valley firm. Married to a successful businessman who spends a lot of time traveling, Ann feels the strain of holding their domestic life together and raising their two daughters, aged three and twelve months. Listen to her as she vacillates between feelings of resentment toward her husband, and guilt that she is

FIGURE 6.1

TOTAL ANNUAL HOURS WORKED, AMERICAN LABOR FORCE PARTICIPANTS

(FROM SCHOR, 1991)

	1969	1987	CHANGE (HOURS) 1969–1987	PERCENT CHANGE
Market Hours				
Men	2054	2152	98	4.7
Women	1406	1711	305	21.7
Household Hours				
Men	621	689	68	10.9
Women	1268	1123	− 145	− 11.4

too demanding of her husband while not doing enough for her children:

> When I come home at six-thirty, take care of the kids, cook dinner, go to bed, get woken up by the baby, I get totally exhausted. I can't stand it anymore. Then I dump on him for not keeping up his fifty percent of the bargain, and causing me to feel so harassed all the time.

> He knows now this is just a phase. During this phase, he tries very hard to come home at six, help with dinner, the bath, and make an equal number of house-related calls.

Then I feel guilty because these errands disrupt his work. His work has always been more important than mine, because he's more talented and more interesting than I am.

But sometimes my wanting-to-protect-him phase only lasts a day. Then I flip back. I say, "I put in almost as many hours. By most people's standards, mine is a respectable position. I'm well paid. I have authority. Just because I don't take my work as seriously as you do doesn't mean other people don't take it seriously. So I only have to do fifty percent at home (p. 105).

Over time, Ann has tried nearly all the strategies that working mothers use. She worked a 7:45 to 6:00 workday and then kept her three-year old daughter up until 8:30 in order to be able to spend more time with her (the "supermom" strategy). She tried outsourcing a good deal of child care to the family baby-sitter, reducing her notion of how much time her children needed to be with her or her husband (the strategy of redefining "needs" at home). She cut back on her mental commitment to work. She cut back time spent with old friends, seeing them only in the context of getting their children together (the strategy of redefining personal needs). The final straw comes when her younger daughter gets sick:

I'm on the verge of quitting. Right now my twelve-month-old daughter is very clingy as a result of an ear infection. She was colicky to begin with and now if I don't hold her, she screams. I'm supposed to go on a business trip tomorrow, and I have a strong urge to say, "I'm not going." I told my husband, but I *can't* tell my boss my child's sick. The worst thing I could possibly do is to acknowledge that my children have an impact on my life (p. 96).

Unable to withstand the pressure of the "second shift," she quits. For working women like Ann Myerson, the time crunch isn't just limited to meeting the demands of child-bearing, childrearing, and housework. Women also take up a disproportionate share of the responsibility of caring for elderly and sick family members, giving rise to the "sandwich" generation caught between raising young families while caring for elderly relatives. Notwithstanding the frequently repeated political rhetoric about the need for policies to "strengthen working families," American workplace provisions for maternity or parental leave are among the stingiest in the industrialized world (Figure 6.2).

FIGURE 6.2

MANDATED PARENTAL LEAVE POLICIES FOR SELECTED INDUSTRIALIZED COUNTRIES

(FROM RESKIN AND PADAVIC)

Country	Duration of Leave (in weeks)	Percentage of Pay	Recipient
Sweden	12–52	90% for 38 weeks	Mother or father
Germany	52	100% for 14–18 weeks	Mother or father
Austria	16–52	100% for 20 weeks	Mother
Italy	22–48	80% for 22 weeks	Mother
Chile	18	100% for 18 weeks	Mother
Canada	17–41	60% for 15 weeks	Mother
U.S.A.	12	0	Mother or father

Sweden's policies are the most generous: 270 days of leave at 90 percent pay after a child's birth, another 90 days at a lower rate of pay, and up to 18 months of unpaid leave. By comparison, parental leave in the United States is paltry. Until very recently, the United States had no federal laws requiring employers to provide any kind of leave (including sick leave), and few employers voluntarily offered it. Then, in 1993, President Clinton signed into law the Family and Medical Leave Act. The act, which applies only to workplaces with fifty or more employees, requires employers to provide up to twelve weeks of unpaid leave and job protection after a pregnancy or other family emergency. Because most American workers work in small businesses, most remain uncovered. Neither is the law of any value to parents who cannot afford unpaid leave. By current estimates, fewer than 40 percent of working women have benefits or income protection that would allow them to take a six-week unpaid leave (Reskin and Padavic, 1994).

SPENDING TIME WITH YOUR LOVED ONES CAN IMPROVE YOUR HEALTH

The time squeeze has far-reaching implications beyond raising the levels of stress, marital discord, and parental guilt: Less leisure time leaves less time for the activities that really make a difference to our well-being, such as spending more time with our families, friends, and neighbors. Over decades of research, social scientists have amassed evidence that suggests that spending time with our loved ones as well as being engaged in social activities are among the surest ways to prolong life and enhance the quality of life (House, et al., 1988). Those who maintain close, confiding relationships with others have been consistently shown to lower their risk of premature mortality. They are also much less susceptible to a host of ailments ranging from common colds, pregnancy complications, depression and attempted suicide, stroke and heart attacks, progression of HIV disease, and even some forms of cancer. Those who engage in a variety of social activities—whether it takes the form of being active in local voluntary organizations or joining church groups—similarly benefit from resistance to illness. A recent Swedish study found that, even after controlling for differences in initial health status and educational attainment, those who took part in frequent leisure-time cultural activities—singing in a choir, attending musical concerts, visiting art exhibitions, going to the cinema and the theater performances, attending sports events as a spectator, and the like—were likely to live significantly longer than those who rarely took part in such activities (Bygren, et al., 1996).

As societies become more absorbed into the global market economy, and leisure time begins to erode, citizens respond by retreating from public life into the private sphere. Individualism becomes exalted, while social bonds weaken and the institutions of the "commons" wither (Seligman, 1990). The result has been a startling rise in the incidence of depressive illness over time. We have entered what the former director of the National Institute of Mental Health (NIMH) dubbed "the age of melancholy" (Klerman, 1979). In a survey of nine industrialized countries across the globe—from North America and Western Europe to Asia and the Pacific Rim—researchers have detected a striking increase in the incidence of depression over time. Not only are people suffering from depression at an earlier age than previously, but those born since World War II are ten times more likely to suffer from depression than those born earlier.

Each succeeding generation since World War II has shown a greater tendency toward depression. A quarter of the American population now experiences depression at least once over the course of their lives (Cross-National Collaborative Group, 1992).

The political scientist Robert Lane draws direct a link between the dramatic rise in depression and the weakening of social bonds caused by the time squeeze and the rise of consumer culture (Lane, 1994). In preindustrialized and less marketized cultures, depression is hardly observed. For instance, among the Kaluli tribe in New Guinea, hopelessness, despair, depression, or suicide are virtually unknown. As recounted by Seligman (1990), if you lose something valuable in this culture, such as your pig, there are rituals (such as dancing and screaming at the neighbor who you think killed the pig) that are recognized by society:

> When you demand recompense for loss, either the neighbor or the whole tribe takes note of your condition and usually recompenses you one way or another. . . . [Thus] the reciprocity between the culture and the individual when loss occurs provides strong buffers against loss becoming helplessness and hopelessness (Seligman, 1990, p. 4).

The insight that depression and suicide are linked to the weakening of social bonds dates all the way back to observations made by the "father of sociology," Émile Durkheim (1897). Comparing suicide statistics in European countries across time and space, Durkheim concluded that the lowest rates of suicide occurred in societies with the highest degrees of social integration. Conversely, an excess of suicides occurred in societies undergoing various forms of dislocation and loosening of social bonds. Though difficult to prove, one might speculate that our overcommitment to work and the increasing amount of time that Americans devote to consumption-oriented activities— shopping and TV watching—have gradually squeezed out the time and attention that people give to social affiliation. Indeed, the political scientist Robert Putnam (1995a; 2000) has convincingly argued that affiliative behaviors of all kinds in American society have been falling at alarming rates since the mid-1960s. For instance, surveys of the time budgets of average Americans in 1965, 1975, and 1985, in which national samples of men and women recorded every single activity undertaken during the course of a day, imply that the time we spend on informal socializing as well as visiting friends and neighbors is down—by as much as one-quarter over the twenty-year period. Similarly, participation in diverse clubs and organizations—from Rotary clubs, the PTA, the Red Cross, the League of Women Voters, and even bowling leagues—is down by roughly 50 percent during the same period (Putnam, 1995b). Some of the most precipitous declines in sociability have occurred during the same period of time that income inequality rose, and Americans have been working longer hours and spending more of their leisure time in front of their television sets. Although considerable controversy was stirred by Putnam's claim that the introduction of television was the principal culprit behind the decline in sociability—a claim that he has subsequently revised (Putnam, 2000)— there can be no doubt that television watching promotes passivity and social isolation, and that in turn, social isolation is a major risk factor for depression.

The connection between social ties and improved health and well-being most likely operates through several distinct mechanisms (Berkman and Glass, 2000). Many of us obtain social support of various kinds—cash loans or child care during an emergency, important new health tips, emotional support during personal crises—from our network of intimate partners, close friends, and contacts. Such support is often indispensable for coping with periods of stress, such as spells of unemployment or major illness, and may make the difference between life and death for individuals and families with few resources.

A follow-up study of heart attack patients found that the availability of emotional support was the strongest predictor of survival, even after taking account of medical factors that determined prognosis (Berkman, et al., 1992). Among patients admitted to the hospital with a heart attack, almost 38 percent of those who reported no source of emotional support died in the hospital compared with 11.5 percent of those with two or more sources of support. The patterns persisted even after patients were discharged. At six months, 52.8 percent of those with no support died compared with 36.0 percent of those with at least one source of support, and 23.1 percent with two or more sources of emotional support. These patterns were remarkably consistent for both women and men, younger and older patients, and those with more or less severe degrees of heart damage.

Turning to breast cancer, Spiegel and colleagues (1989) conducted a clinical trial in which fifty patients with advanced disease were randomly assigned to a weekly support group intervention, and compared with a group of thirty-six patients who received no support-group therapy. Over subsequent follow-up a substantial difference emerged in the survival times in favor of the group who received the support-group therapy.

The mean survival time for the therapy group was 36.6 months compared with 18.9 months for the comparison group.

Lastly, in a series of elegant experiments, Sheldon Cohen and colleagues at the University of Pittsburgh reported exposing a series of volunteers to controlled doses of the common cold virus (Cohen, et al., 1997). In these carefully conducted experiments, the researchers sought to identify the factors that promoted individual resistance. Two hundred and seventy-six healthy volunteers were quarantined in a hotel after they were checked to make sure that they were not already infected with the cold virus. At the end of the first twenty-four hours of quarantine, the researchers deliberately introduced a controlled infectious dose of the common cold virus to the experimental subjects via nasal drops. During the subsequent five-day period of quarantine, experimental subjects were housed individually and told that they could interact with one another but only at a distance of three feet or more. On each day, subjects were checked for the development of cold symptoms, such as a runny nose, cough, sneezing, sore throat, fever, and headache. In meticulous fashion, the researchers went to the extent of measuring nasal mucus production by weighing used tissues on a daily basis. At the beginning of the study, subjects filled out a questionnaire on health habits, as well as their engagement in twelve different types of social relationships—including spouse, parents, parents-in-law, children, other close family members, close neighbors, friends, workmates, schoolmates, fellow volunteers (e.g., charity or community work), members of groups without religious affiliations (e.g., social, recreational, or professional), and membership of religious groups. By the end of the five-day follow-up, over 99 percent were infected with the virus (as detected by the presence of live virus from nasal secretions); however, only about half developed symptoms of cold. The factors that predicted risk of developing a cold included well-established risk factors such as cigarette smoking, lack of sleep, lack of exercise, and taking less than 85 milligrams of vitamin C per day. Strikingly, susceptibility to the cold was also predicted by the size of people's social networks—even though prior theory might have led the researchers to predict that more sociable people would end up with more colds! (Figure 6.3).

Among individuals with fewer than three types of social con-

FIGURE 6.3

SOCIAL NETWORK DIVERSITY AND INCIDENCE OF THE COMMON COLD

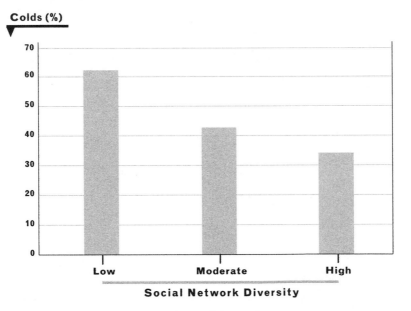

Source: Cohen, et al.

nections, over 60 percent succumbed to the cold, compared with about 40 percent among those with four to five types of connections, and slightly over 30 percent for those with six or more connections. In other words, there was a "dose-response" relation between the diversity of social networks and susceptibility to the cold. Some, but not all of the association, was accounted for by the fact that socially isolated people were more likely to smoke and be less physically active. In short, social networks appeared to influence people's susceptibility to colds by strengthening their immunity to infection (Cohen, et al., 1997).

Space does not permit us to cite the numerous other studies that suggest a link between social affiliation and improved health outcomes. But an influential review article published in *Science* more than a decade ago concluded that the evidence for the health benefits of social ties is as good as that available to the surgeon general in 1964 when he first declared that smoking was a cause of lung cancer (House, et al., 1988).

Even if busy Americans somehow managed to find the time to socialize with their friends and kin, there are still plenty of other commonsense grounds to be concerned about what the time crunch means for our ability to stay healthy. For instance, lack of time is the most commonly cited barrier preventing Americans from engaging in regular exercise, resulting in the present epidemic of sedentary behavior, obesity, diabetes, and hypertension in this society. Many Americans are so busy that their predicament has spawned an industry of personal support services, such as professional grocery shoppers, personal chefs, and dog walkers. Some see the boom in personal services as yet another sign of the increasing polarization in jobs: The rich get richer, while the poor get to run their errands (Bader, 1999). Increasingly, the rich not only delegate those routine daily chores to professionals, but even the very things that form the essence of our social life, such as gift giving (at weddings and Christmas), to choosing a marriage partner. One such businesswoman, operating from Manhattan, charges Wall Street stockbrokers $10,000 for arranging a dozen dates a year. Since 1993, when she incorporated her business, she reports that an active stock market means financial executives spend more time at the office and have less time to find spouses. In the age of declining leisure, even finding a prospective marriage partner, it seems, has turned into "another kind of outsourcing" (Kuczynski, 1999).

The final bastion against outsourcing in our harried lives has been the care and attention we devote to raising our own children. But even here, family values are succumbing to the pressure of the global economy. A kind of "global care chain" has sprung up to replace the time we used to spend raising our children, as documented by the researcher Rhacel Parrenas (and recounted by Arlie Russell Hochschild, 2000). Vicky Diaz (a pseudonym) is a thirty-four-year-old mother of five who emigrated from the Philippines to work as a housekeeper and nanny to the two-year-old son of a wealthy family in Beverly Hills. Though she is college-educated and worked as a travel agent in the Philippines, she realized she could make far more in the United States ($400 per week) than she could back home. Despite her husband's and her own children's misgivings, she became convinced that this was the only way she could afford to raise her own large family. Each week, she sends money back home, including the $40 per week to pay for her own family's live-in nanny back in the Philippines. But the "globalization of mothering" had obviously taken its emotional toll on Vicky. As she told Parrenas:

"Even though it's well paid, you are sinking in the amount of your work. Even while you are ironing the clothes, they can still call you to the kitchen to wash the plates. It was also very depressing. The only thing you can do is give all your love to the child [the two-year-old American child]. In my absence from my children, the most I could do with my situation is give all my love to that child" (quoted in Hochschild, 2000, p. 130).

The "global care chain" is complete when a mother's love for her children becomes commodified, and the resulting "emotional surplus value" is passed on from (a) an older daughter from a poor family in a poor country, who cares for her siblings while (b) her mother works as a nanny caring for the children of an immigrant nanny who, in turn, (c) works as a substitute mother for the child of a family in a rich country.

FAILING TO ACHIEVE THE AMERICAN DREAM: THE COSTS OF SOCIAL EXCLUSION

Earlier, we stressed that spending more on consumer goods, for those who can afford it, does not guarantee more happiness or better health. Instead of getting what we want, working Americans have ended up "wanting what they get" (Schor, 1997).

But what does stepping on the hedonic treadmill mean for the health of individuals near the bottom of the economic heap, who strive hard to buy into the American Dream, yet fall short? The anthropologist William Dressler, of the University of Alabama, has conducted a series of investigations addressing the health consequences of frustrated consumer aspirations. Using a technique in anthropology called "cultural consensus analysis," which involves interviewing key informants, Dressler found that the residents of diverse communities have a single, shared cultural model of what is the acceptable standard of living in such communities (Dressler, 1996). Interestingly, the "acceptable" standard of living turns out not to be one characterized by conspicuous consumption, but more by middle-class standards of comfort in that society, or what Veblen termed a "community-defined standard of decency" (Veblen, 1912). On the other hand, luxury is to a considerable extent a relative concept. The community-defined standard of decency obviously shifts upward with the level of economic development of society, as illustrated by two consensus analyses conducted by Dressler, one in a Brazilian city in the state of São Paulo, and the other in an African-American community of a small southern city (Figure 6.4). Comparing what the respondents at each location deemed as "important" or "not important" to the definition of the successful lifestyle, it is evident that the basket of consumer commodities required to satisfy community standards of decency in American society is both more diverse and luxurious relative to Brazilian tastes. Hence several items deemed "important" by African-Americans—air conditioning, VCR, television—appear under the "not important" list for Brazilians. On the other hand, several items under the "important" column for Brazilians—such as a shower, a bed, or a refrigerator—seem so basic to the American style of life that they were not even mentioned.

According to Dressler, individuals in each society strive to adopt the material style of life that is considered customary for their community. He coined the term "cultural consonance in lifestyle" to refer to the degree to which individuals succeed in

FIGURE 6.4

CONSENSUS RATINGS OF ITEMS RATED AS IMPORTANT OR NOT IMPORTANT IN THE DEFINITION OF THE SUCCESSFUL LIFE

(ADAPTED FROM DRESSLER, 1996 AND 1999)

SÃO PAULO	SOUTHERN CITY, U.S.A.

Items rated important

Shower	New home/home ownership
Refrigerator	Central heat/air conditioning
Gas/Electric stove	Telephone/television
Beds	Car
Dining table	VCR/cableTV
Telephone	Microwave
Automobile	Washer/dryer

Items rated not important

Computer	Stereo
VCR	Computer
Television	Cell phone
Air conditioning	CD player
Motor scooter	Video camera
Expensive house	Belonging to social clubs

achieving the cultural model of lifestyle. To the extent that individuals strive and fail to meet the cultural ideal, adverse health consequences follow. In studies conducted in poor communities in Brazil (1996) and in the United States (1998; 1999),

Dressler and his colleagues demonstrated that the degree of divergence from cultural consonance is associated with higher levels of perceived stress as well as with elevated levels of blood pressure, even though the commodity requirements to satisfy cultural consonance vastly differed between the two cultures. Once again, what seems to matter for health status is not the absolute level of consumption, but one's position in relation to the local standard of living. Neither was the effect of cultural consonance on health trivial. In the African-American sample, for instance, living a lifestyle that was culturally consonant was associated with a 20 percent reduction in the risk of hypertension, even after controlling for differences in income level, occupational status, and educational attainment (Dressler, 1997). Cultural consonance was an even stronger predictor of the risk of hypertension than one's personal level of income.

Further evidence that thwarted aspirations may play a crucial role in the excess levels of high blood pressure among African-Americans come from the studies of so-called John Henryism, conducted by Sherman James of the University of Michigan (James, et al., 1983; James, et al., 1987). According to a black American folk tale, John Henry was a strong but uneducated steel driver who died of exhaustion immediately after he successfully conquered a mechanical steel drill. Sherman James constructed a questionnaire that taps into the extent to which individuals strive hard to succeed in American society. One study of low-income black men in North Carolina found that men who scored high on the John Henryism scale, but had lower-than-average levels of educational attainment, were much more likely to develop high blood pressure (James, et al., 1983). In other words, the active pursuit of material success without the requisite social or economic resources to achieve the American Dream was linked to much higher risk of developing hypertension. Consistent with this theory, African-Americans who had high levels of income or education did not suffer the same risk of hypertension, even if they scored high on the John Henryism scale. In short, there is something toxic about a culture that glorifies material success through hard work but leaves the playing field so tilted that millions are bound to try and end up being cast down.

For those at the very bottom of the economic heap—the so-called urban underclass—who have little or no hope of escaping poverty, crime is sometimes the only recourse for attaining the community standard of living. The sociologist Robert Merton (1968) noted that crime occurs when the high cultural value placed upon competitive achievement clashes with widespread disparities in the actual living standard within society:

> What makes American culture relatively distinctive . . . is that it is a society which places a high premium on economic affluence and social ascent for all its members. . . . This patterned expectation is regarded as appropriate for everyone, irrespective of his initial lot or station in life. . . . This leads to the subsidiary theme that success or failure are results wholly of personal qualities, that he who fails has only himself to blame, for the corollary to the concept of the self-made man is the self-unmade man. To the extent that this cultural definition is assimilated by those who have not made their mark, failure represents a double defeat: the manifest defeat of remaining far behind in the race for success and the implicit defeat of not having the capacities and moral stamina needed for success. . . . It is in this cultural setting that, in a significant portion of cases, the threat of

defeat motivates men to the use of those tactics, beyond the law or the mores, which promise "success.". . . The moral mandate to achieve success thus exerts pressure to succeed, by fair means and by foul means if necessary (Merton, 1968).

Ethnographic work on urban street gangs bear out Merton's theory (Anderson, 1990; MacLeod, 1987; Venkatesh, 1997). In a study based in a public housing project in Chicago, Sudhir Venkatesh (1997) documented how street gangs in the 1980s took over the distribution of crack cocaine with businesslike efficiency. Despite the patent illegality of the drug trade, the motivations of youths who joined such gangs were practically indistinguishable from values endorsed by the American mainstream:

> These are American youths shaped by the same sorts of aspirations that many youths have at that age. Conspicuous consumption is central to their daily lives. They're interested in being mobile. They're very conscious of wanting to be fathers and providers and heads of families. Although gang members feel excluded from American society and act in ways that are violent and counterproductive, they also think of themselves as citizens and want to be citizens (Venkatesh, quoted in Hodder, 1999).

Closely linked to this illegal economy are the deadly outbreaks of violence by which those who are socially excluded regularly express their pent-up frustrations. The rate of violent crime in a society is an exquisitely sensitive mirror of disparities in social conditions. Studies both internationally and within the United

States have found consistent and powerful associations between the extent of inequalities in the material standard of living and the rate of murder (Hsieh and Pugh, 1993; Wilkinson, et al., 1998). Whether we are talking about the soaring rates of homicide in countries like post–Soviet Russia or Venezuela, or the numbing toll of firearm slayings in American cities, wherever social conditions are desperately unequal, violence is sure to occur. This is true in the city of Rio de Janeiro, one of the most unequal cities in one of the most unequal societies in the world. According to analyses carried out by Dr. Celia Szwarcwald and her colleagues at the Oswaldo Cruz Foundation in Rio de Janeiro, it is the degree of income disparity that explains the patterns of homicide across the twenty-six areas of that city, not the poverty rate or the rate of illiteracy (Szwarcwald, et al., 1999). Across American states homicide rates were found to correlate with both income inequality and poverty rates. But income inequality was even more strongly correlated with homicide rates than poverty (correlation coefficients were +0.74 and +0.53, respectively). Even after adjusting for poverty, income inequality accounted for 52 percent of the variance between states (Kawachi, et al., 1999).

Despite the much-touted declines in murder rates within the largest U.S. cities since 1994, our national statistics on homicide still far outstrip other industrialized nations. To put things in perspective, the annual toll of homicides in Britain (population: 58 million) have fluctuated between 700 to 800 in recent years, which puts it in a league with Chicago, a city of less than 3 million (McGuire, 1996). In midsize American cities like Nashville, Cincinatti, Chattanooga, and Louisville, murder rates continue to soar to record levels (Janofsky, 1998).

The American response to our homicide crisis has been to incarcerate everyone, as we noted earlier. But there are limits to the number of new prisons we can build with strapped tax dollars. One predictable result has been the increasingly private solutions that citizens have sought to shield themselves from the waves of crime—by fleeing to gated and secure communities, to which we next turn.

CHAPTER 7

THE SOCIAL COSTS
OF CONSUMPTION

MATERIAL GOODS AND POSITIONAL GOODS

The flip side of consumption is waste. You can tell a lot about a society's material standard of living by observing what gets thrown out in the household garbage. Anecdotally, many visitors to affluent societies like the United States and Japan have been astonished by the sheer quantity and variety of goods that are regularly tossed out on garbage collection day. It is not unusual for indigent individuals living in such societies to depend on practices like "Dumpster diving" for their daily sustenance (Eighner, 1993). Nor is it uncommon to hear stories of hard-up graduate exchange students in Japan sneaking out at night to harvest perfectly usuable pieces of household furniture off the sidewalks, including lamps, vacuum cleaners, and even sofas. Contrast this to a place like Mexico City, where an estimated seventeen thousand garbage-pickers, or *pepenadores,* eke out a meager daily existence by picking through the leftovers of Mexican society—cans, bottles, cardboard, scrap metal, paper, and meat bones (these last destined for manufacturers of bouillon cubes and glue) (Rathje and Murphy, 1992). In desperate places like the Philippines, where one-third of its inhabitants live on less than $1 a day, whole shantytowns have sprung up on garbage dumps. One such dump outside Manila City was featured on the world news in the summer of 2000, when a landslide of garbage buried over two hundred people who were eking out an existence in its shadow. The garbage dump, tragically nicknamed The Promised Land, reached fifty feet high and covered seventy-four acres before its collapse. A whole economy had grown around the heap, with millions of pesos exchanging hands as middlemen bought and resold the salvaged scraps, and shanty shops hawked everything from bicycle parts to school supplies. Like any free-market economy, this one was also characterized by a brutal social hierarchy. At the top of the ladder were owners of junk shops who had contracts with large enterprises, especially hotels, to claim and recycle their garbage. These contractors prepaid for those truckloads and maintained an indentured workforce of scavengers to pick through the garbage. Lower on the social ladder were the freelance scavengers who were forced to comb through the leftover garbage after the choice material had already been picked out. And at the bottom were the "jumpers," who made a precarious living leaping onto the trucks before they dumped, snatching what they could, and often suffering serious injury (Mydans, 2000). A day after the tragic landslide, the scavengers were back to work. Such is the power of raw capitalism.

You can also learn a lot about consumer behavior by systematically rummaging through people's household garbage—

which is exactly what an intrepid group of anthropologists have been doing for two decades in the University of Arizona's Garbage Project (Rathje and Murphy, 1992). In one study carried out between 1986 and 1988, the researchers counted the quantities of hazardous waste that were discarded in the trash of representative households from New Orleans, Phoenix, Tucson, and Marin County, California. As the team sifted though mountains of trash, an interesting pattern emerged: While the proportions of hazardous waste in household garbage did not seem to vary among neighborhoods with sharply different socioeconomic characteristics, the composition of the hazardous waste varied considerably. The hazardous waste from low-income households consisted disproportionately of car-care items: motor oil and gas additives in particular. Middle-income households, in contrast, seemed to lavish less attention on their cars and more on their homes; their hazardous waste consisted disproportionately of paints, stains, varnishes, and various other products dedicated to home improvement. Finally, the garbage emanating from households in affluent neighborhoods reflected the greater attention paid there to lawns and gardens: It contained unusually high amounts of pesticides, herbicides, and fertilizers (Rathje and Murphy, 1992).

People tend to spend a good chunk of their income on consumer products that define their lifestyles. By lifestyles we mean the choices people make with respect to material culture—especially consumer culture—that partially define one's place in the system of social status or prestige (Veblen, 1912; Bourdieu, 1984). Lifestyles serve as indicators of social identity, irrespective of whether they are intended to be conspicuous. Lifestyle consumption is visible and therefore inevitably functions as a sign of social distinction (Bourdieu, 1984). Low-income house-

holds spend money on improving their dearest material possession, the automobile, whereas higher-income households spend
money on improving their most valued asset: the house and
garden.

Returning to the earlier distinction that we drew between material and positional goods, it is clear that auto-care, home-
improvement, and lawn-and-gardening products all fall
predominantly under the latter category of goods, i.e., they are
intended to signal the social position of the purchasers, and
their respective lifestyles involving cars, homes, and gardens. To
sharpen the contrast between material and positional goods,
Hirsch (1976) drew a parallel distinction between "private" and
"social" aspects of consumption. The satisfaction that we obtain from consuming goods that satisfy our material wants is
largely private: "To a hungry man, the satisfaction derived from
a square meal is unaffected by the meals other people eat, or if
he is hungry enough, by anything else they do. His meal is an entirely private affair. In technical terms it is a pure private good."
By contrast, the salient characteristic of social consumption
(and hence, of a positional good) is that the satisfaction individuals draw from them depends not only on their own consumption but on consumption by others as well. The owners of cars,
homes, and gardens may value them for private reasons, but the
satisfaction derived from their use must also be partly social in
nature—otherwise they would not be spending money on improving their outward appearance. Indeed, the profitability of
industry depends on the value that consumers attach to products beyond their instrumental uses. Henry Ford learned this
lesson earlier in the century when he thought he had perfected
the formula for the mass consumption of the automobile—by
selling millions of Model T cars at a small profit to keep prices

low. Unfortunately, his marketing strategy was overtaken by General Motors in the 1920s, who devised a carefully orchestrated campaign that taught consumers to view the automobile as a status symbol, not just as a mode of transportation. Thus, the Chevrolet was pitched for the "hoi polloi," the Pontiac for "the poor but proud," the Oldsmobile for "the comfortable but discreet," the Buick for "the striving," and the Cadillac for "the rich" (Zunz, 1999).

At this point, one might ask what could be the harm in spending money on positional goods. After all, who cares if your neighbor just spent $65 on a copper watering can, or $80 on a designer trowel? If spending more on gardening products encourages your neighbor to contribute toward the beautification of the neighborhood (a positive externality), we might actively encourage it. However, it turns out that not all types of positional spending are so innocent. As Hirsch took pains to demonstrate, some forms of positional spending impose a deadweight loss to society, while others are downright harmful.

POSITIONAL COMPETITION

As we hinted above, many types of goods serve both a private and social function. Even positional goods serve some private function (such as the calorie content of that spoonful of beluga caviar I just swallowed). But the key insight provided by Hirsch's work was to point out that a wide range of private exchanges involve a public-goods element, and that such instances are much more extensive than we routinely allow.

Positional competition—or the quest for relative status— causes us to engage in behaviors that the economist Robert Frank (1999) has dubbed "Smart for One, but Dumb for All."

The conflicts between individual interests (getting more education) and collective interests (preventing credential inflation) are
far more pervasive than most of us realize. For example, young
parents want the best education for their kids, so they end up
working longer and harder to put up that down payment on a
house in a good neighborhood where there is a good public
school (Smart for One). But if everyone else does the same, at
best their relative positions will remain unaffected (since there
are only a limited number of positions in the best schools), and
at worst they merely succeed in driving up housing prices in that
neighborhood (Dumb for All). We each end up with a worse
bargain than was reckoned with before the transaction was undertaken. The invisible hand fails to allocate resources effi-
ciently when there are pervasive individual/group conflicts.
Moreover, Frank contends that such conflict between individual
and group interests is the most important explanation for our
current imbalance in patterns of consumption.

Frank (1999) asks us to engage in a thought experiment:
Imagine two parallel universes identical in every respect except
one. In universe A, everyone lives in houses with four thousand
square feet of floor space, whereas in universe B, everyone lives
in houses with three thousand square feet. Would there be a difference in the well-being of these two universes? Everything we
have learned from psychology tells us there would not: "Rather,
we would expect each society to have developed its own local
norm for what constitutes adequate housing, and that people in
each society would therefore be equally satisfied with their
houses. . . ." (p. 78).

But it takes real resources to build four-thousand-square-feet
houses instead of three thousand-square-feet ones. What, then,
are the opportunity costs of living in the former universe? What

alternative uses could those resources have been put to, that might have improved the well-being of citizens in universe A? Frank's answer is that we have been neglecting the so-called "inconspicuous" forms of consumption—forms of consumption that really make a difference to our well-being—in favor of conspicuous consumption. By inconspicuous consumption, we mean things like improved public infrastructure (e.g., freedom from traffic congestion), more time spent with family and friends, more leisure. As we argued in the previous chapter, each of these types of consumption has been steadily declining in American society. We shall now turn to discuss two examples of consumption in the positional sector with increasingly negative consequences for the welfare of the public: suburban sprawl, and the rise of gated communities.

SUBURBAN SPRAWL

Americans have been fleeing the congestion of cities ever since the 1920s, when, coinciding with the mass marketing of the automobile, those with the money to commute began evacuating the urban centers and moving to the suburbs. The process of suburbanization started in earnest after 1948, when Levitt and Sons undertook the construction of Levittown on Long Island, twenty-three miles from downtown Manhattan. At Levittown, the Levitts "did for the suburban house what Henry Ford did for the automobile" (Moe and Wilkie, 1997). Seventeen thousand homes were built almost overnight to accommodate eighty-two thousand people, a scale of development unprecedented in American history. The houses were built by a streamlined production system, faster and cheaper than anyone had done previously. The pace of suburbanization greatly accelerated during the 1970s and 1980s, financed by local subsidies for development as well as federal tax breaks for real estate construction.

The original attraction of suburban living consisted of its open spaces, cheaper land, and proximity to the countryside, while at the same time allowing residents to live close enough to the city to have access to its jobs and cultural amenities. However, the more suburbs attracted refugees from the city, the less attractive they became. Suburbanization is a classic example of positional competition. It has forced residents to play a form of musical chairs, in which those living in inner cities move to the inner suburbs, forcing those living in inner suburbs to move to the outer suburbs, forcing those living in outer suburbs to move into formerly rural exurbia. "Sprawl" is the term used to describe the hollowing out of cities, and the progressive spread of residential development into the rural hinterland.

Between 1970 and 1990, the population of metropolitan Los Angeles grew by 45 percent, but the land area of the metropolis sprawled by 300 percent. Over the same period, the area of greater Philadelphia grew by 32 percent, even while its population shrank by 3 percent. Metropolitan Cleveland also declined in population while its area expanded by a third. Over the last ten years, the state of Michigan lost 845,000 acres of farmland to suburban development, an area roughly the size of Rhode Island. Since the 1950s, Pennsylvania has lost more than 4 million acres of farmland to suburban sprawl, an area larger than Connecticut and Rhode Island combined (Purdum, 1999).

Conspicuous consumption in the form of ever larger homes—"McMansions"—lies behind the tendency of suburban sprawl to gobble up ever wider tracts of land. Paradoxically, while the size of the average American household has shrunk, the size of the average new house has grown. In 1970, the average size of a new home was 1,500 square feet, but by 1997, it was 2,150 square feet. Because the average household size declined from 3.14 to 2.64 persons over the same period, the average space per person increased from 478 to 814 square feet (Cox and Alm, 1999). Today, 30 percent of new homes in the United States are more than 2,400 square feet, compared with 18 percent in 1986. A typical $750,000 trophy house on the market these days comes with features such as columned entrances, two-story foyers with marble floors, bathrooms with "his" and "her" dressing rooms, three-car garages, double-sized whirlpool tubs, steam showers, home offices, and nanny suites (*San Francisco Business Times,* 1998). It has been pointed out that the average size of a three-car garage (about 700 square feet) is almost as big as an entire first-generation suburban house that was built in Levittown. Take the case of Bill Schweinfurth, chief operating officer of a mobile-home management company, profiled in a magazine article by Linda Baker (2000):

> After moving to Portland from Los Angeles two years ago, the Schweinfurths built a 4,200-square-foot home on their 2-acre lot off Skyline Boulevard. Admitting that they hardly ever use the living and dining rooms, Maggie Schweinfurth says owning a four-bedroom, five-bathroom home is about the little luxuries space affords. Big closets mean she never has to put away off-season clothes; a second laundry room makes washing a breeze. And the bathrooms? "one for the kids, one for the master bathroom, a powder bath for entertaining, and one for the guest room." The only superfluous

not-quite-bathroom, she muses, is off the mud room—the area leading to the backyard. The shower for the dog, she adds, was her husband's idea.

Unfortunately for the rest of us who are unable to afford such displays of conspicuous consumption, these mansions end up inflating land values, squeezing us out of desirable suburbs into ever more remote "exurbs." Even conscientious people who want to do the right thing—build modest, environment-friendly homes—can't afford the price of land.

The growing disparity in the wealth and incomes of Americans is exactly mirrored by the growing divide between "McMansion" mania on the one hand, and the shrinkage of affordable housing on the other. Inequitable housing subsidies and exclusionary zoning laws are partly to blame. For instance, according to the National Low Income Housing Coalition, an estimated 18 percent of housing subsidies in fiscal year 2000 will go to households with an average income of under $9,000. By contrast, an estimated 63 percent of total housing subsidies will go to households with an average income of $123,000 or more. At the same time, zoning regulations in many suburban municipalities are biased toward large homes. Some of our wealthiest suburban neighborhoods establish minimum lot sizes with two-car garages, and limit or outlaw smaller houses and multifamily dwellings (Baker, 2000).

Apart from the environmental degradation caused by sprawl, suburban residents spend ever longer hours commuting to work in congested traffic. Even as our houses continue to grow larger, the average length of our commute to work continues to increase—by 7 percent from 1983 to 1990 (Frank, 1999). Between 1970 and 1989, the number of cars on the road increased by 90 percent, while the urban road capacity grew by less than 4 percent. A ten-mile commute in Los Angeles, which took twenty minutes to complete in 1990, took thirty to thirty-five minutes in 1992—an increase of 50 percent in just two years (Koslowsky, 1998). The Federal Highway Administration predicts that delays during driving time will increase from 2.7 billion vehicle hours in 1985 to 11.9 billion hours by 2005 (Frank, 1999). The costs of commuting are not just measured in the billions of hours of lost productivity—the World Resources Institute estimates that roadway congestion costs $100 billion annually in lost productivity (Hawken, 1997)—but also in terms of the human costs of reduced mental and physical well-being. Besides heightened levels of aggravation ("road rage"), anxiety, and tension associated with commuting, the time or travel distance between home and work has been directly linked with increased blood pressure, secretion of stress hormones, and cold/flu symptoms (Koslowsky, 1998). Ironically, the more families move to the suburbs to escape the congestion of cities, the more they end up battling congested commuter traffic.

But there is altogether another category of cost associated with suburban sprawl, and that is the loss of social cohesion. According to Robert Putnam, every additional ten minutes of commuting cuts community involvement by 10 percent—fewer public meetings attended, fewer church services attended, less volunteering, and so on. In a symbolic sense also, the construction of ever larger trophy homes fuels the resentment and social exclusion of an increasing number of Americans who cannot afford the American Dream. During a decade when the houses of those who could afford them grew bigger, and were inhabited by fewer people, the average rate of home ownership in this country actually declined. Home ownership declined from a peak of 65.6 percent in 1980, to 64.1 percent in 1990 (Newman, 1993). Although small, this downward shift represents the first time in more than fifty years—since the time of the Great Depression—that the rate has fallen. Stagnating incomes among the baby-boom generation contributed to the downward pressure on home ownership. While the construction of upscale housing boomed in the 1980s, the stock of affordable housing—especially single-room-occupancy hotel rooms— virtually disappeared. The number of one-room rental units fell 41 percent between 1985 and 1989 alone, contributing to the rise in homelessness (Jencks, 1994).

The simultaneous rise in the number of suburban mansions and the number of homeless people is a poignant reminder of the decline in social solidarity in this country. As divisions and distances between Americans have widened, so have gaps in mutual aid, social trust, and "social capital" (Moe and Wilkie, 1997). In the previous chapter, we argued that the time bind caused by the cycle of "work and spend" had reduced our level of sociability. We may now add a geographic dimension to the explanation of the disappearance of social capital—the increasing residential segregation of the haves and have-littles (Kawachi and Kennedy, 1997). Of all the forms of residential segregation, the rise of gated communities is perhaps the most pathognomonic.

THE RISE OF GATED COMMUNITIES
Gated communities are residential areas with restricted access in which normally public spaces are privatized. Gated commu-

nities do not simply refer to condominium developments with security systems or doormen. As described by Edward Blakely and Mary Gail Snyder in *Fortress America: Gated Communities in the United States* (1997), the "gates" in such communities can range from:

> ... elaborate two-story guardhouses staffed twenty-four hours a day, to roll-back wrought-iron gates to simple electronic arms. Guardhouses are usually built with one lane for guests and visitors and a second lane for residents who may open the gates with an electronic card, a code, or a remote control device. Some communities with round-the-clock security require all cars to pass the guard, issuing identification stickers for residents' cars. Others use video cameras to record the license plate numbers and sometimes the faces of all who pass through. Entrances without guards have intercom systems, some with video monitors, that residents may use to screen visitors (Blakely and Snyder, 1997; p. 2)

The earliest gated communities in this country appeared in the 1970s in the form of planned retirement developments like Leisure World. Beginning in the 1980s, however, gated communities began to spread to resorts and country club developments, and then to middle-class suburban subdivisions, spurred by the real estate speculation of that decade, as well as rising trends in conspicuous consumption. Now it is estimated that over 4 million Americans live in such gated communities, and they can be found in every major metropolitan area. Currently about one-third of the gated communities are luxury developments for the upper- and upper-middle class; another third are retirement oriented; and the remainder are for the middle class.

The taste for gated communities seems to be growing. A 1990 survey of southern Californian home shoppers found that 54 percent wanted to buy in a gated development (Blakely and Snyder, 1997).

The flight of Americans to gated suburbs is motivated by precisely the social pathologies ascribed earlier to rising income inequality, namely, perceptions of rising crime and the erosion of community cohesion. Safety to walk the streets by day or night, the ability to protect one's property, good services, and infrastructure—these are the commodities that prospective home-buyers seek, and which have become increasingly scarce because of the inability of municipalities to provide them. Sadly, each individual's action to flee from these social pathologies ends up exacerbating them even further for the rest of society. It is a classic instance of a strategy that is "Smart for One, but Dumb for All." We cannot blame gated-community residents for the problems of urban America, or for their efforts to escape the influence of these problems on themselves and their families. Yet the sum of each individual act to remove themselves from the mainstream of society does not correspondingly improve the position of all individuals taken together. There is an "adding-up" problem, because, in essence, the demand for privatized communities is a form of positional competition. To the extent that gated communities actually succeed in shutting out crime, it forces a zero-sum game on the rest of society. What one family gains in protection from property theft, another loses by becoming the new target of crime. If everyone moved to gated communities, this would defeat the ability of such places to deliver safety, exclusiveness, peace, and quiet.

Even the ostensible ability of gated communities to deliver an increased sense of community is likely to be self-defeating.

Many families seek such communities on the assumption that a congregation of similar-minded families within walled boundaries will give rise to a greater spirit of community cohesion. Once they move, however, they may find themselves surrounded by an enclave of individuals who have little interest in contributing to an increase in community spirit—after all, their neighbors must include a self-selected group of individuals who dropped out of society precisely to avoid interacting with others. Empirically, Blakely and Snyder (1997) found in their national study of gated communities that they are no better than society as a whole in producing a strong sense of collective citizenship: "Neighborhood in the sense of a collectively identified boundary can be physically created, but neighborhood in the sense of mutual responsibility is much harder to produce" (p. 135).

In their search for community spirit, many residents of gated communities find paradoxically that their individual liberties become curtailed in ways they did not anticipate. One of the salient features of gated communities is their system of governance, which usually consists of homeowner associations (HOAs). In turn, HOAs come with covenants, conditions, and restrictions that impose rules on a wide-ranging array of things both inside and outside the home. Rules on exterior maintenance are standard, requiring that landscaping conform to a common plan and that houses be painted in a limited number of colors. Pets above a certain size are sometimes barred, as are people under a specific age. There may be height limits on trees and shrubs, approved flower lists. Window air conditioners, backyard swing sets, and satellite dishes are commonly banned. Rules usually forbid hanging the laundry outside, leaving garage doors open, parking campers in driveways, placing trash cans out on the street before a certain hour. In extreme instances, there are restrictions governing home furnishings that can be seen from windows, as well as the hours after which residents may not socialize outside their own houses. In some communities, roving private patrols hand out tickets for parking or speeding violations within the compound (Blakely and Snyder, 1997). Although the ostensible goal of these arrangements may be to reestablish a sense of community solidarity and cohesion, the methods used are often far less communal than controlling. In other words, in seeking out connections to "social capital" in an era of declining sociability, residents of gated communities frequently end up paradoxically paying for the "downsides" of social capital (Portes, 1998).

Perhaps the most deleterious aspect of gated communities is that they may eventually threaten democracy itself. Homeowner associations represent a new form of private government. Financed by private contributions, HOAs provide not only services like landscaping and maintenance of recreational facilities, but also an increasing number of services that municipal governments have abrogated on the grounds of strapped budgets. Such services include garbage pickup, snow removal, streetlights, libraries, and, of course, policing and security systems. It is estimated that in 1992, there were some 150,000 HOAs in the United States, and that their numbers are growing at a rate of 10,000 per year (Blakely and Snyder, 1997). Predictably, paying out of pocket for neighborhood amenities makes residents of gated communities reluctant to part with tax dollars for the general kitty. As Fred Hirsch (1976) wrily remarked: "With a double lock on your door, private guards at the apartment gates, and the private bills all this involves, your enthusiasm for bearing additional taxes to pay for more public policemen is likely to wane" (Hirsch, 1976; p. 90)

HOAs have been actively lobbying state legislatures for property tax rebates to cover the services they pay for and deliver themselves. New Jersey, Texas, Maryland, and Missouri allow for adjustments in local taxes to reflect the self-provided services of HOAs. We are thus faced with a supreme irony: While at the national and state levels the public clamor for less government, at the local level Americans are creating more governance institutions. Such trends have led critics like Robert Reich (1991) to question whether these private governments represent an abandonment of the public realm, a "secession of the successful." Or, in the words of one city official from Plano, Texas, describing the attitudes of gated community residents in his town: "I took care of my responsibility, I'm safe here, I've got my guard gate; I've paid my [homeowner association] dues, and I'm responsible for my streets. Therefore, I have no responsibility for the commonweal, because you take care of your own" (Blakely and Snyder, 1997; p. 140).

Sadly, the demand for gated communities is merely the most conspicuous tip of the iceberg when it comes to recent trends in residential segregation. Accompanying the surge in income inequality in the United States since the mid-1970s, there has been a sharp increase in the spatial concentration of both poverty and affluence. Between 1970 and 1990, the percentage of urban poor Americans living in nonpoor neighborhoods—defined as having poverty rates below 20 percent—declined from 45 percent to 31 percent, while the percentage living in poor neighborhoods (poverty rates between 20 percent and 40 percent) increased from 38 percent to 41 percent. At the very bottom, the share of Americans living in the most distressed neighborhoods (over 40 percent poverty) surged from 17 percent to 28 percent (Massey, 1996). These trends in the spatial concentration of the poor do not tell the story of what happened at the opposite end of the income scale, i.e., among the affluent. According to calculations made by Douglas Massey and Nancy Denton, affluence in American society is even more highly concentrated spatially than poverty. In 1970, the typical affluent American family—defined as having an income level at least four times the poverty rate—lived in a neighborhood that was 39 percent affluent. By 1990, this had increased to 52 percent. In other words, the typical affluent person lived in a neighborhood where more than half the other residents were also rich (Massey, 1996).

Such patterns of segregation are doubly harmful to society. First of all, they are harmful to the poor who are left behind in distressed communities to grapple with the multiple social problems that result from the concentration of disadvantage, including chronic joblessness, the disintegration of the family, crime, teenage pregnancy, and drug abuse (Wilson, 1987). But, second of all, segregation is harmful to society at large because of the erosion of social cohesion that follows, which winds up affecting everyone. We shall turn to examine the wider political costs of diminished social cohesion in the next chapter.

Can we afford to maintain these patterns of segregation as a society? Everything we have learned so far about positional consumption warns us that the process cannot continue forever before a limit is reached; we can run, but sooner or later, the afflictions of inequality will catch up with us. There is a physical limit to suburban sprawl, just as there is a limit to the extent to which individuals and communities can secede from society before the social contract breaks down.

THE ROSETO EFFECT

Though we have argued that the polarization of income and assets has resulted in diminished social cohesion, the reverse is also true: As the depth and breadth of our social bonds have weakened, community tolerance of inequality has risen, as reflected by weakened norms against conspicuous consumption. The less dependent we become on other people's good opinions of us, the weaker become the norms governing conspicuous consumption. Exactly this kind of dynamic was illustrated by the famous case study of the community of Roseto in eastern Pennsylvania (Bruhn and Wolf, 1979).

The small town of Roseto (population 1,600) first came to the attention of the medical researcher Stewart Wolf back in the 1950s. The town posed something of a medical mystery, for despite having roughly the same prevalence of "risk factors" for heart disease—such as cigarette smoking, lack of exercise, overweight, diabetes, and consumption of animal fat—the residents of Roseto suffered less than half the rate of heart attack compared with that of surrounding communities. After many rounds of examining, weighing, bleeding, and interviewing the citizens of Roseto, the researchers could come up with only one thing on which their research subjects seemed to differ conspicuously from people living in surrounding areas: The men and women of Roseto expressed a striking degree of solidarity with their community. There was a strong tradition of helping one's friends as well as friends of one's friends. The social emphasis of the community was on interdependence, which could be traced all the way back to the time when the town had been settled by immigrants who originated from the same village in rural Italy. Going hand in hand with this ethos of mutual aid and solidarity were powerful community norms against conspicuous consumption:

> Proper behavior by those Rosetans who have achieved material wealth or occupational prestige requires attention to the delicate balance between ostentation and reserve, ambition and restraint, modesty and dignity. . . . The local priest emphasized that when preoccupation with earning money exceeded the unmarked boundary it became a basis for social rejection. . . . Rosetan culture thus provided a set of checks and balances to ensure that neither success nor failure got out of hand. . . . During the first five years of our study it was difficult to distinguish, on the basis of dress or behavior, the wealthy from the impecunious in Roseto. Living arrangements (houses and cars) were simple and strikingly similar. Despite the affluence of many, there was no atmosphere of "keeping up with the Joneses" in Roseto, no "putting on the dog" (Bruhn and Wolf, p. 79–82).

Alas, as the younger generation of Rosetans began to move away to seek jobs in neighboring towns, and the community entered the mainstream of American life, the once-tight community bonds that held the town together began to weaken, as did the social taboos against conspicuous consumption. Toward the end of the 1960s, the researchers found a community increasingly preoccupied with materialistic values that accompanied the growing level of affluence:

Women became more concerned about their weight, and several joined Weight Watchers. Men turned to new leisure activities that affluence provided, joining country clubs and initiating a local golf tournament. Some took expensive vacations, visiting Roseto, Italy, and other parts of Europe, went on cruises, or traveled to Las Vegas and fashionable resort areas in New Jersey.

During the decade from 1966 to 1975 many Cadillacs and other expensive cars appeared on Roseto's streets, including a handful of Mercedes-Benzes and even a new Rolls Royce. Several expensive houses costing upwards of $100,000 were built in an area of Washington Township that had recently been annexed to Roseto (Bruhn and Wolf, 1979; p. 110–111).

As the researchers themselves acknowledged, the social disruption stemming from the loosening of social bonds might be applauded as evidence of the pursuit of individuality, standing on one's own feet, and being the master of one's own destiny. On the other hand, as social bonds weakened within the community, the rates of heart attack in Roseto caught up with neighboring towns within the span of a decade. The health advantage that Rosetans originally enjoyed—the so-called Roseto effect—became thus an unexpected casualty of their improved material standard of living, along with rising socioeconomic disparities.

In citing the example of Roseto, we are not advocating that we turn the clock back to an idealized vision of the American community as existed in the past, and famously praised by Alexis de Tocqueville (1835). Few would regard a return to the communities of the 1950s as feasible, or even desirable. Rather, the lesson to be gleaned from the Roseto story is what we have tried to emphasize throughout this chapter—that individual actions to improve their social position do not necessarily "add up" to the welfare of the collective.

RECAPITULATION

Let us summarize our arguments up to this point. The growth record of the United States in recent years has delivered neither happiness nor good health. On the other hand, we have paid an increasingly dear price for the widening inequalities between the rich and poor. The rise in consumer culture and positional competition—as well as the feelings of relative deprivation they engender—have not only created enormous social waste but they threaten the functioning of civil society. The search for social status is enshrined in American culture, yet the very nature of social status (that it is a positional good) dictates that the ensuing competition will take the form of a zero-sum game. Only a limited number of people can be at the top of the heap; for every winner, there must be losers. Combined with the observation that economic development itself leads to a continuous expansion in the commodities required to take part in the mainstream of society, the demand for positional goods is guaranteed to be insatiable. Undoubtedly, these processes occur in all societies regardless of how equitably opportunities and assets happen to be distributed. Nonetheless, we contend that the intensity of positional competition, as well as the social waste associated with it, are likely to be proportionately greater in societies that tolerate wide disparities between the status of the rich and poor. Poor health status, high rates of crime, and the decline of civil society are all symptoms of positional competition carried out to its extreme. Far from attempting to emulate the American example, other countries—both developed and less developed—should heed the lessons of the destructive forces wrought by social inequalities on American society.

CHAPTER EIGHT

POLITICS AND HEALTH

THE POLITICS OF RICH AND POOR

Up to this point we have said little about politics, and the potential links between politics and health. Yet as the great German pathologist Rudolf Virchow (1821–1902) declared over a century and a half ago, "All medicine is politics, and politics is nothing but medicine on a large scale." The kind of society we live in, including the well being of its citizens, is the product of the political process. Politics determine what sorts of policies are pursued by democratic governments—for instance, the choice between policies that give priority to promoting economic growth versus those that emphasize a more egalitarian distribution of national income. Or the choice between more or less government involvement in the economy. Or choices over the size of the welfare state, and the level of social spending to assure basic human security in areas such as education, health, and social safety nets.

Judging by the kinds of policies that have been implemented during the past two decades, it will come as no surprise that American political opinions are shifted far to the right of most other industrialized countries. To give a pertinent example, the political scientist Sidney Verba (1987) surveyed the opinions of "stakeholders" of three countries—Sweden, the U.S.A., and Japan—on the issue of equality. The stakeholders included representatives of the "establishment" (business, labor, and farm leaders), "mediating groups" (intellectuals, the media, and politicians from the left and right), and so-called "challenging groups" (consisting of feminist groups, minority activists, and students). Judged by the pretax distribution of income, Sweden was the most unequal society at the time of the study—more unequal than either the United States or Japan. However, due to the active redistributive policies of the Swedish Social Democratic government, the posttax pattern of income distribution in Sweden was considerably more egalitarian than either Japan or the United States.

The results of Verba's survey indicated that on issues of economic equality, there were vast differences between the opinions of Americans on the one hand, and Swedish and Japanese nationals on the other. For example, reacting to the statement "The government should work to substantially reduce the income gap," no Swedish or Japanese group positioned themselves to the right of Republicans or business groups in the U.S.A. (Verba, et al., 1987) (Figure 8.1).

Even today, after a decade of widening earnings disparities, members of the American labor movement are significantly less favorable toward government action than their European counterparts. Fewer than half of American union members are in favor of the government providing a decent standard of living

FIGURE 8.1

ATTITUDES IN THREE COUNTRIES TOWARD GOVERNMENT MEASURES TO REDUCE INEQUALITY

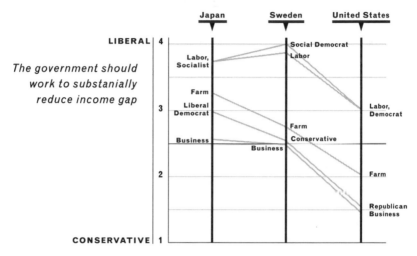

The government should work to substanially reduce income gap

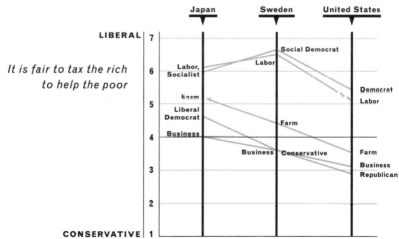

It is fair to tax the rich to help the poor

Source: Verba, et al., 1987

for the unemployed, as compared with 69 percent of West German, 72 percent of British, and 73 percent of Italian unionists (Lipset, 1997). Even the poor in America are inclined to vote against expanding the government's role in providing a decent standard of living for the poor (Figure 8.2).

As evident in Figure 8.2, the proportion of low-income Americans who agree that government has a role in ensuring a decent standard of living for its worst-off citizens is actually *lower* than the proportion of high-income citizens in other European countries who say the same. The extent to which laissez-faire ideals permeate American society has the capacity to occasionally shock even the most stalwart defenders of the free

FIGURE 8.2

ATTITUDES TOWARD GOVERNMENT RESPONSIBILITY IN DIFFERENT AREAS

(FROM LIPSET)

Percent agreeing that government should provide—

	A job for everyone		A decent standard of living for the unemployed		A guaranteed basic income	
	HIGH INCOME	LOW	HIGH INCOME	LOW	HIGH INCOME	LOW
U.S.A.	32	61	23	52	12	33
Great Britain	44	73	57	74	47	71
Germany	77	84	61	72	45	66
Netherlands	60	82	57	68	39	58
Italy	70	93	55	76	53	80

market. Not long ago, New Yorkers learned that the head of their City janitors union was drawing a salary of over $530,000, or about seventeen times what his union members earned on average (Greenhouse, 1999).

Based on the findings of their survey, Verba and colleagues commented that: "The U.S. Government . . . would have trouble launching an ambitious redistributive effort, and few people appear to want it to do so. Americans endorse equality of opportunity [though not outcomes], an ideal that fits well with the individualistic, achievement-oriented principles of free-market capitalism" (Verba, et al., 1987; p. 55). It is a paradox that living in a country with the most clear-cut need of redistributive policies, we remain the least capable of getting them on the political agenda.

Without doubt, part of the explanation of how we got to where we are has to do with deep and long-standing cultural values. The Horatio Alger myth is still alive and well in America. Recent opinion-poll results indicate that almost three-quarters of Americans believe that they have a good chance of improving their standard of living, whereas only about two-fifths of Europeans display the same level of optimism (Lipset, 1997, p. 81). Americans also strongly oppose government restrictions on becoming rich. When the Roper Organization asked the question in 1992, "Do you think there should be a law limiting the amount of money any individual is allowed to earn in a year?" they found that only 9 percent of Americans endorsed such a law, *down* from 24 percent in 1939. The drop was even greater among those at the lowest income level, from 32 to 9 percent (Lipset, 1997; p. 98). Along similar lines, a 1994 survey-based study of "The American Dream," conducted for the Hudson Institute, found that when asked to choose between "having the opportunity to succeed versus having security from failing," an overwhelming 76 percent opted for the former, while only a fifth preferred the security option (Lipset, p. 287).

Still, though the majority of Americans believe in the Horatio Alger myth, economic mobility is not greater in this country than elsewhere, especially for the poor and near poor. For example, measured by the transition rate out of poverty between one year and the next, economic mobility was worse in the United States (13.8 percent) than in France (27.5 percent), Germany (25.6 percent), Ireland (25.2 percent), the Netherlands (44.4 percent), and Sweden (36.8 percent) in the mid 1980s. Only Canada (12.0 percent) had a worse transition rate than the United States—but they also had a lower poverty rate. And measured against the same countries, U.S. low-wage workers are less likely to move into higher-wage jobs (Mishel, et al., 1999).

The perplexing discrepancy between popular attitudes and economic reality can only be reconciled by reference to the American cult of individualism, which abjures government "hand-outs." Our distaste for taxation runs deep in our history and national psyche. From the Boston Tea Party to the Whiskey Rebellion, American history is studded with tax rebellions and armed insurrections against hated taxes (Adams, 1998). To this day, taxes in the United States remain the lowest of all industrialized nations in the OECD (Figure 8.2).

However, Americans are hostile toward taxes not only because we have always been that way, but also because our struggle to maintain ground against the rising tide of income inequality *makes us feel less generous* toward the state. Combined with the pressure to spend more to keep up our social status, we have the perfect formula to ensure there is constant political agitation for tax cuts, as witnessed by the tax rollback revolutions

FIGURE 8.3

GOVERNMENT TAX REVENUE AS A PERCENTAGE OF GDP, 1995

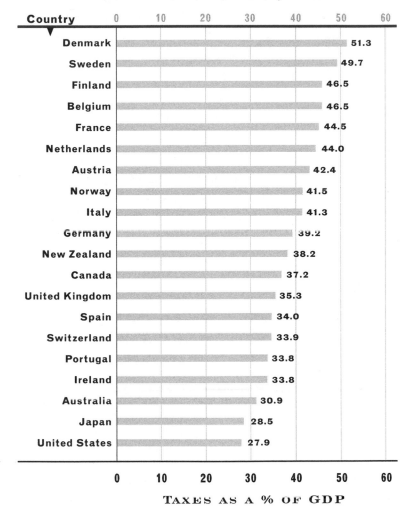

Source: Mishel, et al.

stretching from California (the infamous Proposition 13) to Massachusetts (the equally infamous Proposition 2½) (Newman, 1993, p. 44). The American predicament is in distinct contrast to Europe, where by dint of maintaining higher levels of taxes, citizens tend to view themselves as directly benefiting from government programs—whether in the form of free health care, inexpensive college education, subsidized child care, or better maintenance of public facilities such as mass transportation. As James Galbraith (1998) noted:

> More equal societies will tend to have lower *private* transfer burdens—less private capital, less debt, less conspicuous consumption and pecuniary emulation. People are willing to pay higher taxes for social insurance or they face a lower burden of private debts. Moreover, in a middle-class society, public services come to be seen as collective assets—something from which the population at large benefits directly. What might be a bad social bargain at 30 percent of income, when benefits are thought to flow mainly to the unworthy, seems like a much better deal even at 40 percent of income, when benefits flow back to the population at large (for example, in the form of Canadian medical care, French trains and mass transit, and the German system of free universities (Galbraith, 1998, p. 16).

POLITICAL IDEOLOGY AND HEALTH

In Chapter 3, we argued that population health is linked to income distribution: The more unequal the distribution of income, the lower the health achievement of that society. We may now extend that argument to include the political ideology that gives rise to the pattern of income distribution. The exact pattern of the association between political ideology and population health can be quite complex. At the level of cross-national comparisons, socialist or leftist party participation in national governments is associated with more public spending (Tufte, 1978), higher welfare spending (Hicks and Swank, 1992; Castles, 1982), greater equality in the distribution of income, and ultimately, higher quality of life (Moon and Dixon, 1985). Some studies have found that the more ideologically leftist/socialist the regime, the stronger the role of the state in the economy, and consequently the higher the health achievement of that society. For example, Lena and London (1993) examined whether characteristics of political regimes made a difference to three measures of health—life expectancy, infant mortality, and child death rate—independent of the level of development (gross national product per capita) and international investment dependency (assessed by the extent of transnational corporate penetration). Some eighty-four countries were analyzed, most of them less developed (though some industrial countries like Finland and New Zealand were also included—but not the U.S.A.). As predicted, regimes characterized by a more socialist orientation tended to pursue policies that invested in basic needs, such as improved sanitation, immunization, maternal and child care, nutrition, and housing. These regimes also tended to show significantly lower rates of infant mortality, death among children, as well as higher life expectancy, independent of their level of economic development and investment dependency.

In contrast to cross-national comparisons of political ideology, studies conducted *within* national boundaries reveal that voting patterns are closely linked to health status in the *opposite* direction, i.e., in electoral districts where more people vote for conservative parties, they tend to live longer. Presumably, this pattern is explained by the fact that people living in better circumstances and who have better health are least likely to require public assistance, and hence are also most likely to vote for political parties that promise to dismantle the welfare state. George Davey Smith and Daniel Dorling (1996) analyzed the voting patterns of electoral constituencies in the British elections of 1983, 1987, and 1992. The more voters chose the British Conservative Party, the lower was the mortality rates in their district; conversely, the stronger the showing for the British Labour Party, the worse the health status of that area. As expected, the more deprived the residents of an area (based on measures of car ownership, overcrowded housing, housing tenure, and unemployment), the more they voted for Labour. Even so, the patterns of Conservative/Labour voting were at least as strongly associated with death rates as was the area deprivation measure.

The political culture of a society therefore determines what kinds of policies are pursued by government, and in turn, what kinds of investments are made (or not made) that promote or inhibit health. But that is not the end of the story, for the American predicament cannot be blamed entirely on our history or culture. The fact is that there are systematic biases in the patterns of political participation, which ensure that the voices of the underserved are not transmitted to our elected representatives.

INEQUALITIES IN POLITICAL PARTICIPATION

Participation in political activities provides the mechanism by which citizens in a democracy seek to control who will hold public office and what governments do. Although studies of political participation have tended to focus on voting, there is in fact a whole repertoire of activities by which citizens can engage in politics. These include working in electoral campaigns, contacting government officials, attending protests, working informally with others to solve a community problem, serving without pay on local elected and appointed boards, and contributing money to political causes (Verba, et al., 1995).

Broadening the definition of political participation has important implications for evaluating equality in the political domain. Whereas the act of voting gives equal weight to the preferences of poor and rich citizens, political activities such as giving money are inherently biased toward the rich. During the same period over the last two decades that voter turnout has steadily declined in America, so-called "checkbook participation" in politics has increased. Rapidly rising campaign costs, the increasing role of paid campaign professionals (rather than amateur volunteers), and the development of mass mail and telephone techniques of raising money have all conspired to raise the importance of money-giving as a form of political participation. The net result has been a tilting of the political playing field in favor of the affluent. According to the nationally representative Citizen Participation Survey conducted by the National Opinion Research Center, the richest 3 percent of Americans (with family incomes > $125,000) cast just 4 percent of the votes in the 1988 presidential elections, but accounted for fully 35 percent of all campaign dollars. Meanwhile, at the bottom of the economic hierarchy, the poorest 19 percent of the population (incomes < $14,999) cast 14 percent of the vote, but accounted for only 2 percent of campaign dollars (Verba, et al., 1995). Widening disparities in wealth and income have almost certainly exacerbated this inequality.

In contrast to the skewed patterns of money giving, among individuals who volunteer in political activities the poor are just as likely—if not more likely—to donate their time compared to the rich. Sadly, the influence of voluntarism on the outcome of elections has become steadily overwhelmed by the importance of money. In Congressional elections, candidates who outspend their opponents consistently win. Moreover, voluntarism in the political sphere is itself on the wane due to the erosion of social affiliation described in Chapter 6. The reason is because political activity is embedded in the nonpolitical institutions of civil society. The connection between political participation and civic engagement in voluntary associations can be quite direct, as Verba and colleagues note:

> Social institutions play a major role in stimulating citizens to take part in politics by cultivating psychological engagement in politics and by serving as the locus of recruitment to activity. . . . Ordinary and routine activity on the job, at church, or in an organization, activity that has nothing to do with politics or public issues, can develop organizational and communications skills that are relevant for politics and thus can facilitate political activity. Organizing a series of meetings at which a new personnel policy is introduced to employees, chairing a large charity benefit, or setting up a food pantry at church are activities that are not in and of themselves political. Yet they foster the development of skills that can be transferred to politics (Verba, et al., 1995, p. 17–18).

As citizen participation in voluntary associations wanes, so do the stocks of civic skills that are indispensable for taking part in politics. The more voluntarism declines, the more

importance money assumes in determining the outcome of
politics.

SOCIAL CAPITAL AND POLITICAL PARTICIPATION

Social capital, which we talked about back in Chapter 6, refers to
aspects of social relationships—such as the levels of trust
among citizens, norms of reciprocity, and mutual aid—which
act as resources for individuals and facilitate collective action for
mutual benefit. Social capital represents the resources available
to individuals through their social affiliations and membership
in community organizations. In contrast to financial capital,
which resides in people's bank accounts, or human capital,
which rests in people's heads (via their investment in education
and job training), social capital inheres in the structure and quality of social relationships among individuals. The late sociologist James Coleman (1990) described the manifold forms that
social capital could take. These include moral resources such as
the levels of trust within social relationships, the norms and
sanctions concerning the way that people behave toward one
another, information channels, and so-called "appropriable"
social organizations. As an example of an appropriable social
organization, Coleman cited the case of a residents' association
in an urban housing project that formed initially for the purpose
of pressuring builders to fix various problems—leaks, crum-
bling sidewalks, and so on. After the problems were solved, the
organization remained as available social capital to improve the
quality of life for residents.

The concept of social capital has been applied in a variety of
contexts to explain the ability of communities to solve the

problems of collective action, ranging from the provision of public education to the effective functioning of government institutions. From this brief description, it is evident that Verba and colleagues (1995) are talking about the benefits of social capital when they refer to the "embeddedness of political activity in the non-political institutions of civil society."

According to political scientist Robert Putnam, there is a direct connection between the stocks of social capital in society and the functioning of democracy. His seminal book, *Making Democracy Work* (1993), describes a twenty-year study of a "natural experiment" that took place in Italy in 1970, when central government functions were devolved to local governments for the first time. The subsequent performance of local governments was assessed by a diverse set of policy indicators, including the responsiveness of civic institutions in meeting citizens' needs, as well as measures of the institutions' efficiency in conducting the public's business. The striking conclusion of Putnam's twenty-year study was that stocks of social capital in each region of Italy—as measured by indicators such as the extent of social affiliation, levels of interpersonal trust, and community norms of reciprocity—turned out to be the best predictor of the performance of regional governments. In northern Italy, where citizens actively participate in civic associations—choral societies, soccer leagues, literary guilds, and the like—regional governments were more "efficient in their internal operation, creative in their policy initiatives, and effective in implementing those initiatives" (Putnam, 1993, p. 81). By contrast, in southern Italy, where patterns of civic engagement were much weaker, local government tended to be corrupt and inefficient. Putnam explained his findings in terms of the way social capital enables citizens to cooperate with one another for mutual benefit, and hence overcome the dilemmas of collective action. Reminiscent of Stewart Wolf's decades-long study of the Pennsylvania community of Roseto, citizens living in regions of Italy characterized by high levels of social capital were more likely to trust their fellow citizens, and to value solidarity and equality.

We have argued elsewhere that the same kinds of linkages between social capital and effective participation in democracy may operate across regions of the United States (Kawachi and Kennedy, 1997; Kawachi, et al., 1997; Blakely, et al., 2001). Using the same kinds of social capital indicators that Putnam described in his Italian study namely, membership of voluntary associations, levels of interpersonal trust between citizens, and perceived norms of reciprocity—there turn out to be quite striking geographical variations in the level of social capital across the states of America. In turn, these measures of social capital are correlated with indicators of political participation, such as voter turnout during elections (Figure 8.3). Data on Figure 8.3 were obtained from residents of thirty-nine states sampled in the General Social Surveys conducted by the National Opinions Research Center between 1986 and 1990. Among other questions, the survey asked about membership in a wide variety of voluntary associations—church groups, sports groups, hobby groups, fraternal organizations, labor unions, and so on. The lower the degree of social affiliation—i.e., the more widespread the erosion of social capital—the poorer the voter turnout at election time.

The General Social Surveys also asked questions related to levels of interpersonal trust. Respondents in each state were asked whether they agreed that "most people can be trusted." The correlation of associational membership to interpersonal

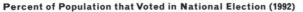

FIGURE 8.4

SOCIAL CAPITAL AND VOTER TURNOUT

Percent of Population that Voted in National Election (1992)

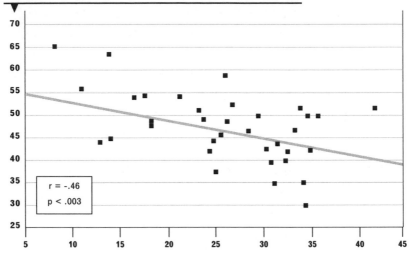

r = -.46

p < .003

**Percent Responding: "Most people would try to take advantage
of you if they got the chance."**

Source: Cohen, et al.

trust was quite high (r = 0.65), and by extension, lack of trust was associated with lower voter turnout.

Disinvestment in social capital is associated not only with aggregate measures of voting, but also with disparities in political participation between the rich and poor. For instance, the lower the levels of trust between citizens, the greater the socioeconomic disparities in participation in political activities of all kinds, including contacting officials, organizing protests, volunteering in campaigns, running for elected office, and so forth.

The obvious question that these kinds of correlations raise is what could account for the marked variations in social capital across American states. According to one account, much of the variation can be explained by historical patterns of immigration and settlement, and long-standing regional differences in political subcultures among the American states. The work of the political scientist Daniel Elazar (1966) is most often cited in this regard. According to Elazar, the political geography of the United States can be divided into three types of political culture: moralistic, traditionalistic, and individualistic. The moralistic political culture most closely resembles the civic culture described by Putnam in northern Italy. Such a culture emphasizes the commonwealth conception as the basis for democratic government. Accordingly, politics is conceived as a public activity centered on some notion of the public good and properly devoted to the advancement of the public interest: "Good government, then, is measured by the degree to which it promotes the public good in terms of the honesty, selflessness, and commitment to the public welfare of those who govern" (Elazar, 1966, p. 90). By contrast, the traditionalistic political culture is rooted in a more paternalistic and elitist conception of the commonwealth: "It reflects an older, pre-commercial attitude that accepts a substantially hierarchical society as part of the ordered nature of things, authorizing and expecting those at the top of the social structure to take a special and dominant role in government" (Elazar, 1966, p. 93). There is a close analogy between Elazar's characterization of traditionalistic culture with the kind of political culture described by Putnam (1993) in southern regions of Italy, where politics tends to be dominated by vertical patron-client relationships as opposed to more "horizontal," egalitarian patterns of political participation observed in the north. Finally, the individualistic political culture tends to emphasize the conception of democracy as a marketplace. In this culture, government is instituted for strictly utilitarian reasons, to handle those functions demanded by the people it is created to serve. Since the individualistic culture emphasizes the centrality of private concerns, "it places a premium on limiting community intervention—whether governmental or nongovernmental—into private activities to the minimum necessary to keep the marketplace in proper working order" (Elazar, 1966, p. 87).

From the foregoing description of Elazar's typology, one would predict that stocks of social capital would tend to be low in regions of America historically dominated by traditionalistic political culture, whereas they would tend to be high in areas characterized by moralistic culture. Using an index of political culture derived from Elazar's typology, this is in fact exactly what we find (Figure 8.5).

Geographically, Elazar's moralistic states are those settled by the Puritans of New England and their Yankee descendants. The Puritans came to America with the intention of establishing the earthly version of the holy commonwealth. Wherever they migrated and settled—first in the New England states, then across the states of the upper Great Lakes, including Michigan, Wisconsin, Minnesota, and Iowa—they established a moralistic political culture. Beginning in the mid-nineteenth century, they were joined by Scandinavians and other northern Europeans who, stemming from a related tradition, reenforced the basic patterns of Yankee political culture. Pressing westward, the Yankees later settled Oregon, then Washington, and were the first "Anglos" to settle California. By contrast, the people who settled the southeastern states sought opportunity in a plantation-centered agricultural system based on slavery:

FIGURE 8.5

ELAZAR-SHARKANSKY POLITICAL CULTURE
INDEX AND SOCIAL CAPITAL (MISTRUST)

Elazar-Sharkansky Political Culture Index

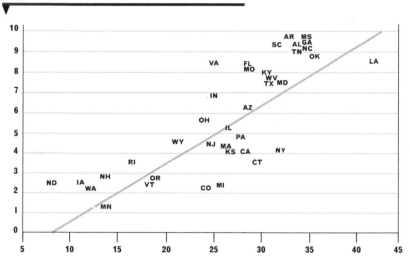

Percent Responding: "Most people would try to take advantage
of you if they got the chance."

This system, as an extension of the landed gentry agrarian-
ism of the Old World, provided a natural environment for
the development of an American-style traditionalistic political culture in which the new landed gentry progressively assumed ever greater roles in the political process at the
expense of the small landholders, while a major segment of
the population, the slaves, were totally excluded from any
political role whatsoever. Elitism within this culture reached
its apogee in Virginia and South Carolina (Elazar, 1966,
p. 102).

The traditionalistic culture was subsequently propagated by settlers into neighboring states: Virginia's people dominated the settlement of Kentucky; North Carolina's influence was heavy in Tennessee; Georgians moved westward into Alabama and Mississippi; and in Louisiana, they mixed with French settlers who shared the same political culture, despite other cultural differences.

Finally, immigrants from England and the interior parts of Germany settled the middle parts of the nation, beginning with the Mid-Atlantic states of New York, New Jersey, Pennsylvania, Delaware, and Maryland. According to Elazar, these diverse groups were united by one common bond—the search for individual opportunity in the New World. Unlike the Puritans who sought communal as well as individualistic goals in their migrations, the pursuit of private ends dominated among the settlers of the middle states. These groups subsequently moved westward into Ohio, Indiana, Illinois, then Missouri.

Thus Elazar's typology, though impressionistic, nevertheless retains a remarkable degree of fidelity in describing the geographic patterns of political culture—and social capital—across the American states. But that is not the end of the story, for the pattern of variation in political culture—established early in the history of the American states—provides an ideal laboratory to examine the influence of social capital on population health outcomes.

SOCIAL CAPITAL AND HEALTH

Just as there are wide geographic variations in the stocks of social capital, so there are marked differences in the health achievement across the American states. When indicators of social capital are arrayed against state differences in mortality and morbidity, the resulting correlations are quite striking. Figure 8.6 shows the relationship between levels of interpersonal trust and the average death rate in the thirty-nine states for which data were available in the General Social Surveys. The lower the level of trust between citizens—as indicated by the proportion of surveyed respondents in each state who believed that "most people cannot be trusted"—the higher is the average death rate.

Similar correlations are obtained when we substitute interpersonal trust with other indicators of social capital, such as the per capita membership of voluntary associations in each state. These relationships occur for mortality among white Ameri-

FIGURE 8.6

THE RELATIONSHIP BETWEEN AGE-ADJUSTED MORTALITY RATES AND LACK OF SOCIAL TRUST

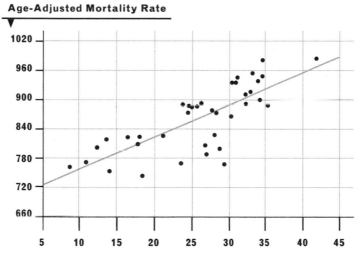

Age-Adjusted Mortality Rate

Percent Responding: "Most people would try to take advantage of you if they got the chance."

FIGURE 8.7

SOCIAL TRUST AND QUALITY OF LIFE

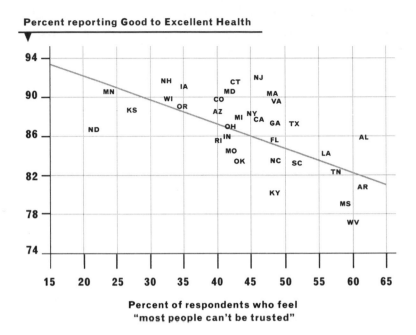

Percent reporting Good to Excellent Health

Percent of respondents who feel "most people can't be trusted"

cans and African-Americans, as well as for both men and women. The correlations are quite robust, and persist after statistical adjustment for state variations in median household income and the proportion of households living below the official poverty threshold (Kawachi, et al., 1997b). Social capital is also correlated with health outcomes other than death rates. For example, Figure 8.7 shows the correlation between the level of interpersonal trust and a measure of self-reported well-being (Kawachi, et al., 1999c). The proportion of residents in each state reporting that their health was only fair or poor (as opposed to good or excellent) was obtained from the Behavioral Risk Factor Surveillance System (BRFSS), carried out by the

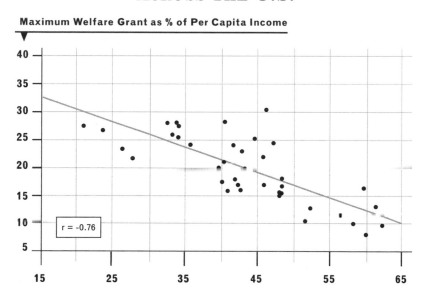

FIGURE 8.8

SOCIAL CAPITAL AND THE LEVEL OF GENEROSITY OF WELFARE GRANTS ACROSS THE U.S.

Maximum Welfare Grant as % of Per Capita Income

r = -0.76

Percent Responding: "Most people can't be trusted."

National Center for Chronic Disease Prevention and Health Promotion. As with mortality rates, a striking correlation is apparent between social capital and quality of life: the lower the level of trust (and also per capita membership of associations), the higher the proportion of citizens who report that their health is poor.

Why should social capital correlate so closely with population health status? At the level of the states, the mechanism seems to be at least partly mediated through inequalities in political participation, which lead to the passage of policies that are systematically biased against the poor. Policy indicators, such as the generosity of welfare benefits, vary systematically with the stocks of social capital in a state (Figure 8.8), and *pari passu,* with the degree of inequality in political participation.

One can imagine that states clustered near the bottom right-hand corner of Figure 8.8 (low levels of social capital, less generous welfare payments) provide a much less hospitable environment for a single mother trying to raise her young children. The social and political culture of these places truncate the range of social opportunities available to the poor, and thereby increase their vulnerability to ill health. The relationship between low political mobilization and adverse social policies has been replicated in other studies. For example, Hill and colleagues (1995) carried out an analysis for the fifty U.S. states from 1978 to 1990, to examine the relationship between the degree of mobilization of lower-class voters at election time, and the generosity of welfare benefits provided by state governments. Even after adjusting for other factors that might predict state welfare policy—such as the degree of pubic liberalism in the state, the federal government's welfare cost-matching rate for individual states, the state unemployment rate and median income, and the state tax effort—the authors found robust relationships between the extent of political participation by lower-class voters and the degree of generosity of state welfare payments. In other words, *who participates* matters for political outcomes, and the resulting policies have an important influence on the opportunities for the poor to lead a healthy life.

The relationships we have discussed are not invariant over time. The importance of state politics and policies wax and wane in response to the broader political climate. For instance, the Reagan and Bush administrations devolved a number of social policy programs to the states, giving state governments an unprecedented degree of control over such policies. At the same time, the 1980s were characterized by major reductions in federal support for social programs, thereby constraining the state lawmakers' ability to respond to voter preferences.

INCOME INEQUALITY AND SOCIAL CAPITAL

Earlier in the book (Chapter 6), we drew attention to the corrosive effects of economic inequality on social affiliation. The more hours people spend at work to keep themselves from slipping backward on the economic ladder the less time they have to volunteer for community activities and to engage in affiliative behaviors of all kinds. Sociability declines as workers expend more hours on the job to bring in the additional income needed to maintain their social position. As the economist Fred Hirsch (1976) put it:

> Friendliness is time consuming and thereby liable to be economized because of its extravagant absorption of this increasingly scarce input. . . . The impact of time pressures on sociability—in the sense of friendliness, social contact, and mutual concern—is made particularly severe by the fact that these relationships do not, by their nature, have the character of private economic goods: which is to say that the costs of benefits of specific actions do not fall primarily on those undertaking them (Hirsch, 1976, p. 78).

The individual choices we make to spend less time socializing with others thus ends up contributing to the decay of the public good we call social capital. If our theory is correct, we would expect that economic inequality is correlated with disinvestment in social capital. That is exactly what we find across the United States (Figure 8.9):

FIGURE 8.9

THE RELATIONSHIP BETWEEN INCOME INEQUALITY AS MEASURED BY THE ROBIN HOOD INDEX, AND LACK OF SOCIAL TRUST

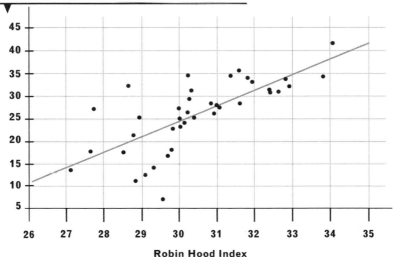

Percent Responding: "Most people would try to take advantage of you if they got the chance."

Robin Hood Index

The horizontal axis on Figure 8.9 displays a measure of income inequality in household incomes across the states, called the Robin Hood index. As the name implies, the Robin Hood index is the proportion of total income that would have to be transferred from affluent to poor households in order to achieve equal distribution of incomes. The more unequal the distribution of income, the lower the degree of social capital as measured by an indicator such as the level of trust among citizens. Much the same degree of correlation would have been obtained had we substituted other forms of social capital on the vertical axis, such as the per capita membership in civic organizations, or the level of perceived norms of mutual aid and reciprocity.

Harking back to the case study of the Italian-American town of Roseto mentioned in the last chapter, civic ties were also observed to weaken there as the community entered the economic mainstream of American society and income disparities widened. Community informants began to complain about declining membership in their civic associations. Although Roseto continued to maintain a higher density of civic associations compared with neighboring towns throughout the three decades of the study, fully 40 percent of Rosetans (compared with a third of those in neighboring Bangor) reported that their organizations had deteriorated or lost members over time. Whereas homes in Roseto used to be built with porches facing the neighbors across the street, beginning in the 1960s, new houses started to appear with porches attached at the back, overlooking private yards. The erosion of civic life in Roseto exactly coincided with the decade during which the rate of heart attack in Roseto caught up with neighboring towns (Wolf and Bruhn, 1993).

Though we have argued that scarcity of time leads to a decline in community commitment, economic inequalities may lead to the erosion of social capital for other obvious reasons. Simply put, the greater the social distance between the incomes of the rich and poor, the greater will be the degree of mistrust between citizens. As a counterweight to the claim that economic inequality promotes the smooth functioning of society by acting as an incentive for greater work effort, the sociologist Melvin Tumin warned many years ago that: "to the extent that inequalities in social rewards cannot be made fully acceptable to the less privileged in a society, social stratification systems function to encourage hostility, suspicion and distrust among the various segments of society and thus to limit the possibilities of extensive social integration" (Tumin, 1953). If the rich and poor share no common economic and social reality, the inevitable consequence is the erosion of trust, solidarity, and social cohesion, as well as little or no agreement on common social goals or vehicles for achieving these goals (Smeeding, 1998).

We referred earlier to the reluctance of Americans to part with tax dollars. Growing inequalities in income surely exacerbate this cultural predisposition. Unfortunately, the more the interests of the rich begin to diverge from those of the typical family, the more this translates into pressure to lower taxes for the rich, and to reduce social spending on the poor. Between 1980 and 1995, the effective federal tax rate for a middle-class family of four hardly changed at all, from 23.7 percent (in 1980) to 24.4 percent (in 1995). By contrast, the average federal tax rates changed substantially for those with the highest incomes. Between 1977 and 1985, changes in the tax laws reduced the tax bill for the wealthiest 1 percent of families by an average of $97,250 per family. Meanwhile, the same revision in the tax code increased the tax payments of the bottom 80 percent of families by an average of $221. Although progressive tax changes in 1986 and 1993 partially reversed some of these inequities, the net reduction in the tax bills of the richest 1 percent still fell by $36,710 since 1977 (Mishel, et al., 1999).

Conservatives like to point out that most of the surge in income inequality described earlier in the book is pretax, i.e., it reflects what employers are putting into paychecks, not what the government is taking out. On the other hand, there can be no gainsaying that the tax policies of the 1980s exacerbated the growth of income inequality in this country. And while tax cuts were partly responsible for the surge in inequality during the 1980s, the reverse is also true of their aftermath: The perception that one is slipping back on the income ladder makes everyone anxious to have their taxes cut back.

In May 2001, President Bush signed into law a ten-year $1.35 trillion tax cut. A majority of Americans expressed approval for some form of tax cut, even as they continued to support the expansion of government programs such as prescription-drug benefits, investment in public education, and shoring up Social Security. These tax cuts will trigger another seismic shift in the distribution of incomes in American society, in favor of the very wealthy. Independent analyses indicate that 40 percent of the benefits of the Bush tax cut will accrue to the richest one percent of taxpayers. The bottom 80 percent will receive less than a third of the benefits, while the bottom 20 percent will get less than 1 percent.

CHAPTER NINE

CONCLUSION

No matter what their level of material comfort or standard of living, Americans want more. We want to shop more and spend more to acquire an ever-expanding list of necessities and "must-have" items. But what does all this extra consumption *get us,* in the end? Have Americans' lives been improved—for example, are we happier or healthier—as a result of all our consumption and accumulation? The arguments in this book cast doubt on this assumption. Unfortunately, the American brand of turbo-capitalism seems to be rapidly catching on in the rest of the world.

For the first time in history, the whole planet is now either capitalist or highly dependent on capitalist economies (Castells, 2000). The collapse of the Soviet Union left no other worldwide rival for capitalism. Replacing the old competition between central planning and capitalism, what emerged from the end of the Cold War has been a struggle for survival among different kinds of capitalism—American, European, Japanese, and Chinese (Gray, 1998). Increasingly, it appears to be one particular strain of capitalism, based on the American model, that is set to take over the rest of the world. This strain of capitalism is much more virulent, as well as more ruthless and volatile compared with the more controlled and regulated capitalism of the 1950s and 1960s. As Will Hutton and Anthony Giddens (2000) describe it:

> Its overriding objective is to serve the interests of property owners and shareholders, and it has a firm belief, effectively an ideological one, that all obstacles to its capacity to do that—regulation, controls, trade unions, taxation, public ownership, etc.—are unjustified and should be removed. Its ideology is that shareholder value must be maximized, that labor markets should be "flexible" and that capital should be free to invest or disinvest in industries and countries at will. It's the capitalism of both Wall Street and financial markets and of street trading and street markets: the capitalism at which the Anglo-Saxon community, and the Americans in particular, have been very good (Hutton and Giddens, 2000, p. 9–10).

As the world has become more "globalized," countries both rich and poor have been forced to adapt to the demands of this new turbocapitalism. Sovereign governments are confronted with a dwindling set of options to implement ambitious countermeasures to head off the threats of foreign competition, speculative capital movements, and looming recessions. Each day, an estimated $1.2 trillion worth of transactions takes place in foreign exchange markets alone—more than the *annual* GDP of a country like France, and considerably more than the total foreign exchange reserves of the world's central banks. Around 95 percent of these transactions are speculative in nature, many using complex derivative financial instruments that threaten the stability of national economies (Gray, 1998). The worldwide mobility of capital and production has resulted in a competitive downgrading of the regulatory and welfare systems of sovereign states. Humane capitalist economies have been forced to deregulate, roll back the welfare state, bully labor into becoming more "flexible." Fiscal conservatism has become the order of the day.

It is a process described by John Gray (1998) as a variant of Gresham's Law, which states that "bad money drives out good money, but good money cannot drive out bad money." In the global free market, bad capitalism drives out the good, in a race to the bottom:

> In any competition that is arranged with rules of global laissez-faire [based on the American model], the social market economies of Europe and Asia are at a systematic disadvantage. They have no future unless they can modernize themselves by deep and rapid reforms.

It would be a mistake to suppose that the present strain of capitalism is a natural product of social evolution—or as Gray (1988) puts it, "a natural state of affairs that comes about when political interference with market exchange has been removed." As Gray remarks, free markets are just as much a product of artifice, design, and political coercion as central planning ever was: "It is an end-product of social engineering and unyielding political will." The coercive element of global capitalism was nowhere as starkly illustrated as during the aftermath of the Asian economic crisis of 1997. Once the crisis struck, the countries involved (Indonesia, Thailand, Korea) found their policies largely dictated by the twin enforcers of the new global economic order: the International Monetary Fund and the U.S. Treasury. The IMF imposed literally hundreds of conditions on these countries as part of their bailout packages. The conditions heaped upon countries in financial crisis typically included drastic measures to ensure debt repayment, such as spending cuts on education and health, elimination of subsidies for basic foods, fuel, and transportation, devaluation of national currencies to make exports cheaper, and privatization of national assets. Some 200 million "newly poor" citizens were minted as a consequence of the IMF's mismanagement of the Asian financial crisis. After the IMF advised these countries to "export their way out of the crisis," the dumping of Asian steel in U.S. markets resulted in the layoffs of over twelve thousand steelworkers (Global Exchange, 2000).

On other occasions, the IMF has been known to impose free-market rules on poor countries that are not even observed in rich, donor countries. Thus, in the 1990s, the government of Haiti was told to eliminate statutes in its labor code that mandated increases in the minimum wage when inflation exceeded 10 percent. By the end of 1997, Haiti's minimum wage was only $2.40 a day, just one-fifth of the minimum wage in 1971 in real terms. Haiti was also forced to open its market to highly subsidized U.S. rice at the same time that the IMF prohibited Haiti from subsidizing its own farmers. A U.S. corporation, Early Rice, now sells nearly 50 percent of the rice consumed in Haiti, with the result that Haitian farmers have been forced off their land to seek work in sweatshops (Global Exchange, 2000).

What does this brand of capitalism augur for the future of the world? As champions of the market are fond of pointing out, the new brand of turbocapitalism has proved extraordinarily effective at keeping inflation down and creating shareholder value. This is good news if you happen to be one of the shareholders. But the vast majority of the world's population toils under the influence of global capitalism without enjoying most of its benefits. Some 85 percent of humankind live outside the developed world, yet the so-called "emerging markets" represent only about 7 percent of global value in market capitalization. Even in the United States, the richest nation in the world, the new economy has left millions of households behind, to struggle in poverty, or worse, locked behind bars. The growing inequality that accompanied the recent economic boom is perfectly captured by the following paradox: nearly one in five Americans are now classified as clinically obese, at the same time as 31 million people (including one in six children) face chronic hunger in any given year.

As the year 2000 drew to a close, the Office of the New York State Comptroller estimated that $15 billion—roughly the size of the gross domestic product of Cuba—was handed out in bonuses to investment bankers on Wall Street, up from $11.9 billion a year before. That translated into an $88,000 bonus for each of the 170,400 workers on Wall Street, except most of the money went to the top. As many as 4,000 senior executives brought home $1 million in bonuses, while the top one hundred deal makers each made more than $10 million (Valdmanis, 2000).

As everybody knows, the story was different in 2001. Due to the downturn in business, year-end bonuses on Wall Street were considerably lower compared to the year before. Nonetheless, executives still took home $10 billion for Christmas. Despite a sharp drop in stock prices (especially after September 11) the Dow Jones industrial average still hovered around 10,000 at year's end.

Meantime, growing queues of children and their newly laid-off parents formed at city food pantries, while the murder rate started to climb again. The social health of the nation—which was already stagnant during the economic *good* times—looked set to take a dive. Yet as Congress debated alternative measures to rescue the economy, was any thought being given to reviving the social health of the nation? Sadly, the kinds of measures debated by our politicians (such as tax breaks for corporations and wealthy individuals) would likely exacerbate our social problems, based on the evidence we have discussed in this book.

Why do we continue to allow market interests to ride roughshod over social considerations? Why do we continue to neglect the state of the nation's social health? Quite simply, the answer may be because Americans are ignorant about the dismal state of our nation's health. Indicators of our social well-being are not fed back to the public in the same manner that myriad market indicators are used to signal the state of the nation's economy on a daily basis.

Consider how we have become quite accustomed to receiving every news or social event accompanied by a running commentary on how the markets reacted. Witness how every twist and turn of the 2000 presidential election was appended by breathless network TV commentary on how the markets responded. Indeed, it is now well nigh impossible to escape the intrusion of the market in our daily lives. Anyone who has taken a flight longer than forty minutes' duration between any city within the northeast is reminded of this fact as the latest Dow

Jones numbers flash across the LCD screen of the air-phones affixed to the cabin seats. Yet in stark contrast to the continual intrusion of the markets in our daily consciousness, scant attention is devoted to our nation's social progress. No news service thinks of following up a report on market performance with a commentary on trends in homicide rates, suicide rates, or infant mortality.

To redress this woeful imbalance, Marc Miringoff and colleagues at the Fordham Institute for Innovation in Social Policy have been working for some years to develop a composite index of the nation's social health. This index, composed of sixteen separate indicators, measures our social performance in areas such as infant mortality, child abuse, teenage drug abuse, and violent crime (Figure 9.2).

As Figure 9.2 demonstrates, our nation's social performance used to track market performance until the late 1970s, at which point it slipped behind, and has stagnated since. It is true that in more recent years, some indicators have improved, such as the teen birth rate, the violent crime rate, and the high school dropout rate. Yet others have worsened, or remained in the doldrums, such that the disconnect between market performance (the Dow Jones Index is now above 10,000) and social performance continues to widen (Miringoff, et al., 1996).

The idea that the American model should be a universal model for the rest of the world to emulate has been a recurrent theme in our national discourse. Yet the wisdom of such a triumphalist notion is plainly cast in doubt by the social price we pay for doing things "the American way." Nor is our claim to be a universally applicable model accepted by the rest of the world: "The costs of American economic successes include levels of social division—of crime, incarceration, racial and ethnic con-

FIGURE 9.1

INDEX OF SOCIAL HEALTH

(FROM MIRINGOFF AND MIRINGOFF, 1999)

AGE GROUP	INDICATOR
Children	Infant mortality
	Child abuse
	Child poverty
Youth	Youth suicide
	Teenage drug abuse
	High school droputs
	Teenage births
Adults	Unemployment
	Wages
	Health care coverage
Elderly	Poverty, aged 65+
	Life expectancy, aged 65+
All Ages	Violent crime
	Alcohol-related traffic fatalities
	Affordable housing
	Inequality

flict and family and community breakdown—that no European or Asian culture will tolerate" (Gray, 1998). There is a social limit to building fortress communities, to sacrificing longer hours on the job, and to mortgaging our collective future on escalating consumption. Sooner or later, we are bound to reach a limit on the number of new prisons we can build, or the pro-

FIGURE 9.2

INDEX OF SOCIAL HEALTH AND THE
DOW JONES INDUSTRIAL AVERAGE,
1970–1993

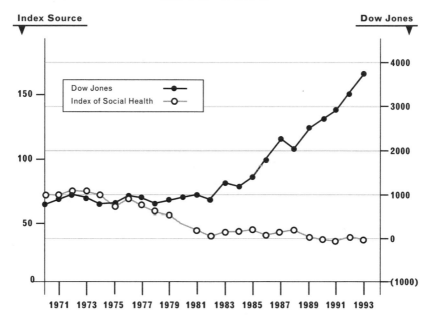

Sources: Fordham Institute for Innovation in Social Policy;
Statistical Abstract of the United States; Survey of Current Business

portion of the underclass we can incarcerate. In the long run, our present behavior is unsustainable, either for the nation or for the planet. Future historians may look back on the American model of capitalism, and legitimately question what it accomplished in the way of advancing human freedoms and capabilities. Market forces, unleashed from social and political control, have a corrosive impact on social cohesion. As Nancy Folbre (2001) has argued, the "invisible hand" of the market threatens to undermine the "invisible heart" of caring, values of reciproc-

ity, and obligation that bind our families and communities together.

Above all, there can be no more convincing demonstration
of the limitations of the American model than the way it com-
promises the health and well-being of our own body politic.
The lackluster performance of our national health indicators
ought to be the occasion for national soul-searching. We make
up just 4 percent of the world's population, yet we expend about
half of all the money spent on medical care (Bezruchka, 2001).
Even so, we rank near the bottom of what Stephen Bezruchka
dubbed the "Health Olympics." In 1970, the U.S.A. ranked
about fifteenth in the world in indicators like life expectancy and
infant mortality. Twenty years later, our position had slipped to
about twenty-second, or just about near the bottom of the
Health Olympics, behind almost all rich countries and a few
poor ones. Not coincidentally, disparities in income and wealth
vastly increased during this same period, even though the *average*
national income continued to rise. Japan, by contrast, started
out near the bottom (twenty-third) of the Health Olympics in
1960, but overtook the rest by 1977 (Bezruchka, 2001). While
the Japanese economy remains in a slump, their health status
continues to rank number one in the Health Olympics. Granted,
there is little to admire about the state of the Japanese economy;
on the other hand, neither has our recent economic expansion
contributed to an improvement in the health of all Americans.

Some people maintain that life expectancy, infant mortality,
and other health indicators *have* improved, on average, over the
years, even though our ranking in the Health Olympics may
have slipped and the disparities in health across the socioeconomic divide have widened. If the average trend is improving,
why fuss about our relative national performance and persistent

gaps between the rich and poor? As Dr. Pangloss remarked in Voltaire's *Candide,* do we not live in the best of all possible worlds? The answer, of course, depends on who you happen to be. If you happen to be an Asian-American woman born in Westchester County, New York, you can indeed expect to live to the ripe old age of 90.3 years, according to the Harvard Global Burden of Disease Project (Murray, et al., 1998). On the other hand, if you happen to be born an African-American male in the District of Columbia, you can expect to live 57.9 years—or lower than the life expectancy of the male citizens of Ghana (58.3 years), Bangladesh (58.1 years), and Bolivia (59.8 years). If you happen to have been a white American, your life expectancy improved, on average, throughout the 1980s and into the 1990s. On the other hand, if you happened to be an African-American, your life expectancy slid backward during the period when income inequality widened in U.S. society (Figure 9.3).

Although the foregoing examples only present the data in black and white, this is partly an artifact of the way official U.S. health statistics are kept. The National Center for Health Statistics is incapable of reporting health statistics by class because data in this country do not happen to be collected in that way (some Marxists have argued that this reflects deliberate government policy). Nonetheless, since race is an (imperfect) proxy for socioeconomic status, the data for black Americans provide some clue about what has been happening to the health of disadvantaged segments of U.S. society during the most recent period of widening economic inequalities. More to the point, the arguments we have marshaled in this book suggest that laissez-faire and unbridled competition threaten the health of us all. No society can indefinitely put off paying for the consequences of relentless competition, escalating consumption, plus all the

FIGURE 9.3

U.S. LIFE EXPECTANCY AT
BIRTH, 1984–1992

(FROM WILLIAMS)

YEAR	WHITE	BLACK
1984	75.3	69.5
1985	75.3	69.3
1986	75.4	69.1
1987	75.6	69.1
1988	75.6	68.9
1989	75.9	68.8
1990	76.1	69.1
1991	76.3	69.3
1992	76.5	69.6

social divisions and social exclusion that the American model of capitalism implies.

Will global laissez-faire turn out to be another twentieth-century utopia, as John Gray (1998) has argued, soon to be swallowed into the memory hole of history? If prosperity cannot deliver sustainable advances in freedoms for all members of society, then what reasons do we have to value economic growth? The answer to *that* question, we submit, has profound implications for the survival of our mode of running the economy, indeed of the globe.

REFERENCES

Aaron, H. J. *Politics and the Professors: The Great Society in Perspective.* Washington, D.C.: Brookings Institution, 1978.

Acocella, Nicola. *The Foundations of Economic Policy: Values and Techniques.* Cambridge: Cambridge University Press, 1998.

Adams, Charles. *Those Dirty Rotten Taxes: The Tax Revolts That Built America.* New York: The Free Press, 1998.

Adler, Nancy E., Thomas Boyce, Margaret A. Chesney, Sheldon Cohen, Susan Folkman, Robert L. Kahn, S. Leonard Syme. "Socioeconomic Status and Health: The Challenge of the Gradient." *American Psychologist* 49 (1994):15–24.

Anderson, Elijah. *Street Wise.* Chicago: University of Chicago Press, 1990.

Anderson, Gerry F., and J. P. Poullier. "Health Spending, Access, and Outcomes: Trends in Industrialized Countries." *Health Affairs* 18(3) (1999):178–192.

Andrews, Edmund L. "Germany's Retailers Beckon Warily to Customers." *The New York Times,* November 2, 1996.

Bader, Jenny L. "Relying on the Competence of Strangers." *The New York Times,* April 1, 1999: D1.

Baker, Linda. "McMansion Mania." *Utne Reader Online.* September 19, 2000, 5 pp.

Becker, B. E., and M. A. Huselid. "The Incentive Effects of Ournament Compensation Systems." *Administrative Science Quarterly* (1992): 37:336–350.

Bell, Quentin. *On Human Finery.* London: The Hogarth Press, 1976.

Berkman, Lisa F., L. Leo-Summers, and Ralph I. Horwitz. "Emotional Support and Survival Following Myocardial Infarction: A Prospective Population-Based Study of the Elderly." *Annals of Internal Medicine* 1992: 117:1003–9.

Berkman, Lisa F., and Thomas Glass. "Social Integration, Social Networks, Social Support, and Health." In: Lisa F. Berkman and Ichiro Kawachi, (eds). *Social Epidemiology.* New York: Oxford University Press, 2000, pp. 137–73.

Bezruchka, Stephen. "Is Our Society Making You Sick?" *Newsweek,* February 26, 2001: p. 14.

Blakely, Edward J., and Mary Gail Snyder. *Fortress America: Gated Communities in the United States.* Washington, D.C.: The Brookings Institution, 1997.

Blakely, Tony A., Bruce P. Kennedy, and Ichiro Kawachi. "Socioeconomic Inequality in Voting Participation and Self-Rated Health." *American Journal of Public Health* (2001): 91:99–104.

Bloom, David E., and David Canning. "The Health and Wealth of Nations." *Science* (2000): 287:1207–1209.

Bloom, Matt. "The Performance Effects of Pay Dispersion on Individuals and Organizations." *Academy of Management Journal* (1999): 42(1):25–40.

Bloom, Matt, and John G. Michel. "The Relationships Among Organizational Context, Pay Dispersion, and Managerial Turnover." *Academy of Management Journal* (2000) in press (can be accessed at: www.aom.pace.edu/amj/unassigned/bloom.pdf).

Blumberg, Paul. *Inequality in an Age of Decline.* Oxford: Oxford University Press, 1980.

Bourdieu, Pierre. *Distinction: A Social Critique of the Judgement of Taste.* Cambridge: Harvard University Press, 1984.

Bradshaw, York W., and Michael Wallace. *Global Inequalities.* Thousand Oaks, CA: Pine Forge Press, 1996.

Brickman, P., D. Coates, R. J. Janoff-Bulman. "Lottery Winners and Accident Victims: Is Happiness Relative?" *Journal of Personality and Social Psychology* (1998): 36:917–927.

Bruhn, John G., and Stewart Wolf. *The Roseto Story: An Anatomy of Health.* Norman, OK: Oklahoma University Press, 1979.

Bryant, Adam. "American Pay Rattles Foreign Partners." *The New York Times,* January 17, 1999, p. 1.

Butterfield, Fox. "Number of Inmates Reaches Record 1.8 Million." *The New York Times,* September 15, 1999.

Bygren, Lars O., Boinkum B. Konlaan and Sve-Erik Johansson. "Attendance at Cultural Events, Reading Books or Periodicals, and Making Music or Singing in a Choir as Determinants for Survival: Swedish Interview Survey of Living Conditions." *British Medical Journal* (1996): 313:1577–80.

Castells, Manuel. "Information Technology and Global Capitalism." In: Will Hutton and Anthony Giddens (eds). *Global Capitalism.* New York: The New Press, 2000.

Castles, Francis. *The Impact of Parties.* Beverly Hills: Sage, 1982.

Center on Budget and Policy Priorities. "Poverty Rate Fails to Decline as Income Growth in 1996 Favors the Affluent." Washington, D.C., 1997.

Citro, Constance F., and Robert T. Michael (eds). *Measuring Poverty: A New Approach.* Washington, D.C.: National Academy Press, 1995.

Cucheo, Steve. "Statistically Speaking, What's Going on in Consumer Bankruptcy?" *ABA Banking Journal* (1997): 89(8):31–2.

Cohen, Sheldon, William J. Doyle, David P. Skoner, Bruce S. Rabin, and Jack M. Gwaltney. "Social Ties and Susceptibility to the

Common Cold." *Journal of the American Medical Association* (1997): 277:1940–1944.

Coleman, James S. *Foundations of Social Theory*. Cambridge: Harvard University Press, 1990.

Cowherd, D. M., and D. I. Levine. "Product Quality and Pay Equity Between Lower-Level Employees and Top Management: An Investigation of Distributive Justice Theory." *Administrative Science Quarterly* (1992): 37:302–320.

Cox, W., Michael and Richard Alm. *Myths of Rich & Poor. Why we're better off than we think*. New York: Basic Books, 1992.

Crocker, David A. "Consumption, Well-Being, and Virtue." In: Neva R. Goodwin, Frank Ackerman, and David Kiron (eds). *The Consumer Society*. Washington, D.C.: Island Press, 1997.

Cross-National Collaborative Group. "The Changing Rate of Major Depression: Cross-National Comparisons." *Journal of the American Medical Association* (1992): 268:3098–105.

Csikszentmihalyi, Mihaly. "If We Are So Rich, Why Aren't We Happy?" *American Psychologist* (1999): 54(10):821–827.

Davey Smith, George, Martin J. Shipley, Geoffrey Rose. "Magnitude and Causes of Socioeconomic Differences in Mortality— Further Evidence from the Whitehall Study." *Journal of Epidemiology and Community Health* (1990): 44:265–270.

Davey Smith, George, David Blane, Mel Bartley. "Explanations for Socioeconomic Differentials in Mortality. Evidence from Britain and Elsewhere." *European Journal of Public Health* (1994): 4:131–144.

Davey Smith, George and Daniel Dorling. " 'I'm All Right, John': Voting Patterns and Mortality in England and Wales, 1981–92." *British Medical Journal* (1996): 313:1573–7.

Davis, Kingsley, and Wilbert E. Moore. "Some Principles of Stratification." *American Sociological Review* (1945): 10:242–249.

Diderot, Denis. *Rameau's Nephew and Other Works*. New York: Bobbs-Merrill, 1964.

Diener, Ed, Jeff Horwitz, and Robert A. Emmons. "Happiness of the Very Wealthy." *Social Indicators* (1985): 16:263–274.

Diener, E., E. Sandvik, L. Seidlitz, M. Diener. "The Relationship Between Income and Subjective Well-Being: Relative or Absolute?" *Social Science Indicators Research* (1993): 28:195–223.

Diener, Ed, and Mary Beth Diener. "Happiness: Subjective Well-Being." In: *Encyclopedia of Mental Health.* Howard S. Friedman (ed). San Diego: Academic Press, 1998.

Diener, Ed. "Subjective Well-Being. The Science of Happiness and a Proposal for a National Index." *American Psychologist* (2000): 55(1):34–43.

Drentea, P. and P. J. Lavrakas. "Over the Limit: The Association Among Health, Race and Debt." *Social Science and Medicine* (2000): 50(4):517–529.

Dressler, William W. "Culture and Blood Pressure: Using Consensus Analysis to Create a Measurement." *Cultural Anthropology Methods* (1996): 8:6–8.

Dressler, William W. "Culture and Patterns of Poverty" Paper presented at the 1997 Annual Meeting of the Society for Applied Anthropology, March 4–9, Seattle, WA.

Dressler, William W, Mauro Campos Balieiro, Jose Ernesto Dos Santos. "Culture, Skin Color, and Arterial Blood Pressure in Brazil." *American Journal of Human Biology* (1999): 11:49–59.

Dressler, William W. "Stress and Hypertension in the African-American Community." Proceedings of the conference on "Public Health in the 21st Century: Behavioral and Social Science Contributions," May 7–9, Atlanta, GA.

Durkheim, Emile (1897). *Suicide.* Ed. George Simpson, transl. J. A. Spaulding and G. Simpson. New York: The Free Press, 1951.

Eaker, Elaine D., Joan Pinsky, and William P. Castelli. "Myocardial Infarction and Coronary Death Among Women: Psychosocial Predictors from a 20-Year Follow-up of Women in the Framingham Study." *American Journal of Epidemiology* (1992): 135:854–64.

Easterlin, Richard. "Will Raising the Incomes of All Increase the Happiness of All?" In: N. R. Goodwin, F. Ackerman, D. Kiron (eds). *The Consumer Society*. Washington, D.C.: Island Press, 1997.

Egan, Timothy. "War on Crack Retreats, Still Taking Prisoners." *The New York Times*, February 29, 1999, p. 1.

Ehrenberg, R. G. and M. L. Bognanno. "The Incentive Effects of Tournaments Revisited: Evidence from the European PGA Tour." *Industrial and Labor Relations Review* (1990) 43:74S–88S.

Elazar, Daniel J. *American Federalism: A View from the States*. New York: Thomas Y. Crowell Company, 1966.

Eighner, Lars. *Travels with Lizbeth*. New York: St. Martin's Press, 1993.

Ekins, Paul. "A Sustainable Consumer Society: A Contradiction in Terms." *International Environmental Affairs* (Fall 1991): 4(4):244.

Faux, Jeff, and Larry Mishel. "Inequality and the Global Economy." In: Will Hutton and Anthony Giddens (eds). *Global Capitalism*. New York: The New Press, 2000.

Filatki, H. and J. Fox. "Differences in Mortality by Housing Tenure and by Car Access." *Population Trends* (1995): 81:27–30.

Flegg, A. T. "Inequality of Income, Illiteracy and Medical Care as Determinants of Infant Mortality in Underdeveloped Countries." *Population Studies* (1982): 36:441–458.

Folbre, Nancy. *The Invisible Heart: Economics and Family Values*. New York: The New Press, 2001.

Frank, Robert H. *Choosing the Right Pond: Human Behavior and the Quest for Status*. New York: Oxford University Press, 1985.

Frank, Robert H. and Philip J. Cook (1995). *The Winner-Take-All Society*. New York: The Free Press, 1995.

Frank, Robert H. *Luxury Fever: Why Money Fails to Satisfy in an Era of Excess*. New York: The Free Press, 1999.

Freeman, Richard B. *When Earnings Diverge: Causes, Consequences, and Cures for the New Inequality in the U.S.* Washington D.C.: National Policy Association Report #284, 1997.

Galbraith, James K. *Created Unequal: The Crisis in American Pay.* New York: The Free Press, 1998.

Galewitz, Phil. "Forbes 400 Net Worth Tops $1 Trillion." *The Washington Post,* September 24, 1999 (can be accessed at: www.wash ingtonpost.com/wp-srv/business/daily/sept99/forbes24.htm).

Garrett, Laurie. *Betrayal of Trust: The Collapse of Global Public Health.* New York: Hyperion, 2000.

Global Exchange Staff (2000). "Top Ten Reasons to Oppose the IMF." www.geocities.com/walrys95482/eagle2-april.html.

Goodwin, Neva R. Volume Introduction. In: Neva R. Goodwin, Frank Ackerman, and David Kiron (eds). *The Consumer Society.* Washington, D.C.: Island Press, 1997.

Gottschalk, Peter, and Timothy M. Smeeding. "Cross-National Comparisons of Earnings and Income Inequality." *Journal of Economic Literature* (1997) XXXV: 633–687.

Gray, John. *False Dawn: The Delusions of Global Capitalism.* New York: The New Press, 1998.

Greenhouse, Steven. "Finding out How Much the Boss Really Makes." *The New York Times,* March 14, 1999.

Hacker, Andrew. *Money: Who Has How Much and Why.* New York: Scribner, 1997.

Hafner, Katie. "Everything but a Dial." *The New York Times,* January 28, 1999: E1, E6.

Hagerty, Michael R. "Social Comparisons of Income in One's Community: Evidence from National Surveys of Income and Happiness." *Journal of Personality and Social Psychology* (2000): 78(4): 764–771.

Hawken, Paul. "Natural Capitalism." *Mother Jones,* March/April, 1997, p. 48.

Herbert, Bob. "Working Harder, Longer" (op-ed). *The New York Times,* September 4, 2000, p. A19.

Hicks, Alexander M. and Duane H. Swank. "Politics, Institutions, and Welfare Spending in Industrialized Democracies, 1960–82." *American Political Science Review* (1992): 86(3): 658–74.

Hill, Kim Q., Jan E. Leighley and Angela Hinton-Andersson. "Lower-class Mobilization and Policy Linkage in the United States." *American Journal of Political Science* (1995): 39(1):75–86.

Hirsch, Fred. *Social Limits to Growth*. Cambridge, MA: Harvard University Press, 1976.

Hochschild, Arlie. *The Second Shift: Working Parents and the Revolution at Home*. New York: Viking Penguin, 1989.

Hochschild, Arlie Russell. "Global Care Chains and Emotional Surplus Value." In: Will Hutton and Anthony Giddens (eds). *Global Capitalism*. New York: The New Press, 2000.

Hodder, Harbour Fraser. "Street Gangs Inc." *Harvard Magazine*, March–April: 14–18, 1999.

House, James S., Karl R. Landis, Debra Umberson. "Social Relationships and Health." *Science* (1988): 214:540–545.

Hsieh, C. C., M. D. Pugh. "Poverty, Income Inequality, and Violent Crime: A Meta-analysis of Recent Aggregate Data Studies." *Criminal Justice Review* (1993): 18, 182–202.

Hutton, Will and Anthony Giddens (eds). *Global Capitalism*. New York: The New Press, 2000.

Inglehart, Ronald. *Culture Shift in Advanced Industrial Society*. Princeton, NJ: Princeton University Press, 1990.

James, Sherman, S. Hartnett, and W. Kalsbeek. "John Henryism and Blood Pressure: Differences Among Black Men." *Journal of Behavioral Medicine* (1983): 6:259–278.

James, Sherman, David Strogatz, Steven Wing, and D. Ramsey. "Socioeconomic Status, John Henryism, and Hypertension in Blacks and Whites." *American Journal of Epidemiology* (1987): 126:1273–1281.

Janofsky, Michael. "Some Midsize Cities Miss Trend as Drug Deals and Killings Soar." *The New York Times,* January 15, 1998.

Jencks, Chrisopher. *Rethinking Social Policy: Race, Poverty, and the Underclass*. Cambridge: Harvard University Press, 1992.

Jencks, Christopher. *The Homeless.* Cambridge: Harvard University Press, 1994.

Judge, Kenneth. "Income Distribution and Life Expectancy: A Critical Appraisal." *British Medical Journal* (1995): 311:1282–1285.

Kahn, Robert S., Paul H. Wise, Bruce P. Kennedy, and Ichiro Kawachi. "State Income Inequality, Household Income, and Maternal Mental and Physical Health: Cross-Sectional National Survey." *British Medical Journal* (2000): 321:1311–5.

Kaplan, George A., Elsie Pamuk, John W. Lynch, R. D. Cohen, Jennifer L. Balfour. "Income Inequality and Mortality in the United States: Analysis of Mortality and Potential Pathways." *British Medical Journal* (1996): 312:999–1003.

Kasser, Tim, and Richard M. Ryan. "Further Examining the American Dream: Differential Correlates of Intrinsic and Extrinsic Goals." *Personality and Social Psychology Bulletin* (1996): 22(3): 280–287.

Kaufman, Leslie. "Luxury's old guard, battered by new realities." *The New York Times,* December 16, 2001.

Kawachi, Ichiro, and Bruce P. Kennedy. "Health and Social Cohesion: Why Care About Income Inequality?" *British Medical Journal* (1997): 314:1037–1040.

Kawachi, Ichiro, Bruce P. Kennedy, Kimberly Lochner, and Deborah Prothrow-Stith (1997b). "Social Capital, Income Inequality, and Mortality." *American Journal of Public Health* (1997): 87: 1491–1498.

Kawachi, Ichiro, Bruce P. Kennedy, and Roberta Glass (1999a). "Social Capital and Self-Rated Health: A Contextual Analysis." *American Journal of Public Health* (1999): 89:1187–1193.

Kawachi, Ichiro, Bruce P. Kennedy, Richard G. Wilkinson (1999b). "Crime: Social Disorganization and Relative Deprivation." *Social Science and Medicine* (1999): 48(6):719–731.

Kawachi Ichiro, Bruce P. Kennedy, Richard G. Wilkinson (1999c).

Income Inequality and Health: A Reader. New York: The New Press, 1999.

Kennedy, Bruce P., Ichiro Kawachi, Deborah Prothrow-Stith. "Income Distribution and Mortality: Cross-Sectional Ecological Study of the Robin Hood Index in the United States." *British Medical Journal* (1996): 312:1004–1007. See also erratum, *British Medical Journal* (1996): 312:1253.

Kennedy, Bruce P., Ichiro Kawachi, Roberta Glass, and Deborah Prothrow-Stith. "Income Distribution, Socioeconomic Status, and Self-Rated Health: A U.S. Multi-Level Analysis." *British Medical Journal* (1998): 317:917–21.

Keynes, John Maynard. *Essays in Persuasion.* New York: W.W. Norton & Company, 1931 (reprinted 1961).

Kilborn, Peter T. "Charity for Poor Lags Behind Need." *The New York Times,* December 12, 1999, p. 1.

Kloby, Jerry. *Inequality, Power and Development: The Task of Political Sociology.* Atlantic Highlands, NJ: Humanities Press, 1997.

Koslowsky, Meni. "Commuting and Mental Health." In: *Encyclopedia of Mental Health.* Howard S. Friedman (ed). San Diego: Academic Press, 1998.

Kozol, Jonathan. *Savage Inequalities: Children in America's Schools.* New York: Harper Perennial, 1991.

Krueger, David W. *Emotional Business: The Meanings of Work, Money and Success.* San Marcos, CA: Avant Books/Slawson Communications, Inc., 1992.

Kuczynski, Alex. "Running Cupid's Wall Street Office." *The New York Times,* February 14, 1999, p. 11.

Kunst, Anton. "Cross-National Comparisons of Socioeconomic Differences in Mortality." Dissertation. Rotterdam: Erasmus University, 1997.

Landes, David S. *The Wealth and Poverty of Nations: Why Some Are So Rich and Some So Poor.* New York: W. W. Norton & Co., 1998.

Lane, Robert E. "Does Money Buy Happiness? A New Look at Income and Utility." *The Public Interest,* Fall, 1993: 56–65.

Lane, Robert E. "Friendship or Commodities? The Road Not Taken: Friendship, Consumerism, and Happiness." *Critical Review* (1994): 8(4):521–554.

Lena, Hugh F. and Bruce London. "The Political and Economic Determinants of Health Outcomes: A Cross-National Analysis." *International Journal of Health Services* (1993): 23(3):585–602.

Leonhardt, David and Riva D. Atlas. "Locking Up the Plastic: Many Americans Cut Back on High-interest Debt." *The New York Times,* October 18, 2001.

Lewin, Tamar. "Gifts to Charity in U.S. Topped $203 Billion in 2000, Study Says." *The New York Times,* May 24, 2001.

Lipset, Seymour Martin. *American Exceptionalism: A Double-Edged Sword.* New York: W. W. Norton and Company, 1997.

Lochner, Kimberly, Elsie Pamuk, Diane Makuc, Bruce P. Kennedy, and Ichiro Kawachi. "State-Level Income Inequality and Individual Mortality Risk: A Prospective, Multi-Level Study." *American Journal of Public Health* (2001): 91:385–91.

Lynch, John W., George A. Kaplan, Elsie R. Pamuk, Richard D. Cohen, K.E. Heck, Jennifer L. Balfour, Irene H. Yen. "Income Inequality and Mortality in Metropolitan Areas of the United States." *American Journal of Public Health* (1998): 88(7):1074–80.

Macintyre, Sally, Anne Ellaway, Geoff Der, Graeme Ford, Kate Hunt. "Do Housing Tenure and Car Access Predict Health Because They Are Simply Markers of Income or Self Esteem?" A Scottish study. *Journal of Epidemiology and Communiy Health* (1998): 52:657–664.

MacLeod, Jay. *Ain't No Makin' It: Leveled Aspirations in a Low-Income Neighborhood.* Boulder, CO: Westview Press, 1987.

McDonough, Peggy M., Greg J. Duncan, David Williams, James House. "Income Dynamics and Adult Mortality in the United

States, 1972 through 1989." *American Journal of Public Health* (1997): 87:1476–1483.

McGuire, Stryker. "The Dumblane Effect." *Newsweek*, October 28, 1996, p. 46.

Massey, Douglas S. "The Age of Extremes: Concentrated Affluence and Poverty in the Twenty-First Century." *Demography* (1996): 33:395–412.

Menzel, Peter. *Material World: A Global Family Portrait.* San Francisco, CA: Sierra Club Books, 1994.

Merton, Robert K., and A. S. Rossi. "Contributions to the Theory of Reference Group Behavior." In: R. K. Merton and P. F. Lazarsfeld (eds). *Continuities in Social Research.* New York: The Free Press, 1950.

Merton, Robert K. *Social Theory and Social Structure.* New York: The Free Press, 1968.

Miringoff, Marc, and Marque-Luisa Miringoff. *The Social Health of the Nation: How America Is Really Doing.* New York: Oxford University Press, 1999.

Miringoff, Marque-Luisa, Marc Miringoff, and Sandra Opdycke. "The Growing Gap Between Standard Economic Indicators and the Nation's Social Health." *Challenge,* July–August, 1996, 17–22.

Mishan, E. J. *Technology and Growth: The Price We Pay.* New York: Praeger Publishers, 1969.

Mishel, Lawrence, Jared Bernstein, and John Schmitt (eds). *The State of Working America, 1998–99.* Ithaca, New York: Cornell University Press, 1999.

Moe, Richard, and Carter Wilkie. *Changing Places: Rebuilding Community in the Age of Sprawl.* New York: Henry Holt and Company, 1997.

Moon, B. E. and W. J. Dixon. "Politics, the State, and Basic Human Needs: A Cross-National Study." *American Journal of Political Science* (1985): 29:661–94.

Mydans, Seth. "Before Manila's Garbage Hill Collapsed: Living Off Scavenging." *The New York Times,* July 18, 2000, p. A6.

Myers, David G. and Ed Diener. "Who Is Happy?" *Psychological Science* 6(1) (1995):10–19.

Myers, Dowell, and Jennifer R. Wolch. "The Polarization of Housing Status." In: Reynolds Farley (ed). *State of the Union: America in the 1990s. Volume One: Economic Trends.* New York: Russell Sage Foundation, 1995.

Newman, Katherine S. *Declining Fortunes: The Withering of the American Dream.* New York: Basic Books, 1993.

Newsweek, "Busy Around the Clock," July 17, 2000, p. 49.

The New York Times. "Fed Says Economy Increased Net Worth of Most Families," by Richard W. Stevenson, January 19, 2000: A1 and C6.

The New York Times. "A Rising Tide, But Some Boats Rise Higher Than Others," by Steven Greenhouse, September 3, 2000: WK 3.

The New York Times. "Personal Spending Rises as Savings Rate Hits a Low." August 29, 2000: C2.

Portes, Alejandro. "Social Capital: Its Origins and Applications in Modern Sociology. *Annual Reviews of Sociology* (1998): 24:1–24.

Purdum, Todd S. "Suburban 'Sprawl' Takes Its Place on the Political Landscape." *The New York Times,* February 6, 1999.

Putnam, Robert D. (1995a). "Bowling Alone: America's Declining Social Capital." *Journal of Democracy* (1995): 6:65–78.

Putnam, Robert D. (1995b). "Tuning In, Tuning Out: The Strange Disappearance of Social Capital in America." *Political Science and Politics* December (1995): 664–693.

Putnam, Robert D. *Bowling Alone.* New York: Simon & Schuster, 2000.

Rathje, William, and Cullen Murphy. *Rubbish! The Archaeology of Garbage.* New York: HarperCollins Publishers, 1992.

Reich, Robert B. (1991). *The Work of Nations: Preparing Ourselves for 21st Century Capitalism.* New York: A. A. Knopf, 1991.

Reskin, Barbara, and Irene Padavic. *Women and Men at Work.* Thousand Oaks, CA: Pine Forge Press, 1994.

Revkin, Andrew C. "Welfare Policies Alter the Face of Food Lines." *The New York Times,* February 26, 1999a, p. 1.

Revkin, Andrew C. "As Need for Food Grows, Donations Steadily Drop." *The New York Times,* February 27, 1999b, p. A17.

Rodgers, G. B. "Income and Inequality as Determinants of Mortality: An International Cross-Section Analysis." *Population Studies,* (1979): 33:343–351.

Rozhon, Tracie. "The Card-Carrying Angst of the Dysfunctional Shopper." *The New York Times,* December 20, 1998.

Schembari, James. "A Price Not Paid in Money." *The New York Times,* March 2, 1999.

Schor, Juliet B. "New Analytic Bases for an Economic Critique of Consumer Society." In: N. R. Goodwin, F. Ackerman, D. Kiron (eds). *The Consumer Society.* Washington, D.C.: Island Press, 1997.

Schor, Juliet B. *The Overworked American: The Unexpected Decline of Leisure.* New York: Basic Books, 1991.

Schor, Juliet B. *The Overspent American: Upscaling, Downshifting, and the New Consumer.* New York: Basic Books, 1998.

Segal, Jerome. "Alternatives to Mass Consumption." *Philosophy and Public Affairs* (special issue on Ethics of Consumption). (Fall 1995): 15(4): 27–29, 276.

Seligman, Martin E. P. "Why Is There So Much Depression Today? The Waxing of the Individual and the Waning of the Commons." In: R. E. Ingram (ed). *Contemporary Psychological Approaches to Depression.* New York: Plenum Press, 1990: pp. 1–9.

Sen, Amartya. *Inequality Re-examined.* Cambridge: Harvard University Press, 1992.

Sen, Amartya. "Mortality as an Indicator of Economic Success and Failure." *The Economic Journal,* (1998): 108:1–25.

Shapiro, Isaac. "Unequal Shares: Recent Income Trends Among the

Wealthy." Washington, D.C.: Center on Budget and Policy Priorities, November, 1995.

Shapiro, Isaac and Robert Greenstein. "The Widening Income Gulf." Washington, D.C.: Center on Budget and Policy Priorities, 1999 (can be accessed at: www.cbpp.org/9-4-99tax-rep.htm).

Smeeding, Timothy M. "U.S. Income Inequality in a Cross-National Perspective: Why Are We So Different?" In: James A. Auerbach and Richard S. Belous (eds). *The Inequality Paradox: Growth of Income Disparity.* Washington, D.C.: National Policy Association, 1998, pp. 194–217.

Smith, Adam (1759). *The Theory of Moral Sentiments.* London: Bell, 1907.

Solnick, Sara J., and David Hemenway. "Is More Always Better? A Survey on Positional Concerns." *Journal of Economic Behavior and Organization* (1998): 37:373–383.

Spiegel, David, J. R. Bloom, H. C. Kraemer, and E. Gottheil. "Effect of Psychosocial Treatment on Survival of Patients with Metastatic Breast Cancer." *Lancet* (1989): 2:888–91.

Starfield, Barbara. *Primary Care: Balancing Health Needs, Services, and Technology.* New York: Oxford University Press, 1998.

Stouffer, A. E., E. A. Suchman, L. C. DeVinney, et al. *The American Soldier Volumes I and II.* Princeton, NJ: Princeton University Press, 1949.

Swarns, Rachel L. "Future Threatens a Place without Calendars." *The New York Times,* January 1, 2000: A5.

Szwarcwald, Celia Landmann, Francisco Inacio Bastos, Francisco Viacava, and Carla Lourenco Tavares de Andrade. "Income Inequality and Homicide Rates in Rio de Janeiro, Brazil." *American Journal of Public Health* (1999): 89:845–850.

Tangcharoensathien, V., P. Harnvoravongchai, S. Pitayarngsarit, and V. Kasemsup. "Health Impact of Rapid Economic Change in Thailand." *Social Science and Medicine* (2000): 51:789–807.

Tocqueville, Alexis de (1835). *Democracy in America.* New York: Vintage Books, 1945.

Thurow, Lester C. and Robert E. B. Lucas. "The American Distribution of Income: A Structural Problem." U.S. Congress, Joint Economic Committee, March 17, 1972. Quoted in: Hirsch, Fred. *Social Limits to Growth.* Cambridge: Harvard University Press, 1976, p. 51.

Tufte, Edward. *The Political Control of the Economy.* Princeton, NJ: Princeton University Press, 1978.

Tumin, Melvin. "Some Principles of Stratification: A Critical Analysis." *American Sociological Review* (1953): 18:387–394.

Uchitelle, Louis. "As Taste for Comfort Rises, So Do Corporations' Profits." *The New York Times,* September 14, 1997, pp. 1 and 34.

United Nations Development Program. *Human Development Report 1998.* New York: Oxford University Press, 1998.

Valdmanis, Thor. "Bonuses Mean Investment Bankers Don't Need Regis." *USA Today,* November 20, 2000, B1.

Veblen, Thorstein. *The Theory of the Leisure Class.* New York: Penguin, 1912.

Venkatesh, Sudhir. "The Social Organization of Street Gang Activity in an Urban Ghetto." *American Journal of Sociology* (1997): 103(1):82–111.

Verba, Sidney, S. Kelman, Gary R. Orren, et al. *Elites and the Idea of Equality.* Cambridge: Harvard University Press, 1987.

Verba, Sidney, Kay Lehman Schlozman, Henry E. Brady. *Voice and Equality: Civic Voluntarism in American Politics.* Cambridge: Harvard University Press, 1995.

Vogel, Shawna. *The Skinny on Fat.* New York: W. H. Freeman, 1999.

Waldman, R. J. "Income Distribution and Infant Mortality." *The Quarterly Journal of Economics.* November, 1992: 1283–1302.

Wallace, Deborah, and Rodrick Wallace. *A Plaque on Your Houses:*

How New York Was Burned Down and Public Health Crumbled. New York: Verso, 1998.

Wennemo, I. "Infant Mortality, Public Policy, and Inequality—A Comparison of 18 Industrialised Countries 1950–85." *Sociology of Health and Illness* (1993): 15: 429–446.

Wilkinson, Richard G. "Income Distribution and Life Expectancy." *British Medical Journal* (1992): 304: 165–168.

Wilkinson, Richard G. "Income and Mortality." In: *Class and Health: Research and Longitudinal Data.* R. G. Wilkinson (ed). London: Tavistock, 1986.

Wilkinson, Richard G. "The Epidemiological Transition: From Material Scarcity to Social Disadvantage?" *Daedalus* (1994): 123: 61–77.

Wilkinson, Richard G. *Unhealthy Societies: The Afflictions of Inequality.* London: Routledge, 1996.

Wilkinson, Richard G. "Health Inequalities: Relative or Absolute Material Standards?" *British Medical Journal* (1997): 314: 591–5.

Wilkinson, Richard G., Ichiro Kawachi, Bruce P. Kennedy. "Mortality, the Social Environment, Crime and Violence." *Sociology of Health and Illness* (1998): 20(5):578–597.

Williams, David R. "Race and Health: Trends and Policy Implications." In: James A. Auerbach and Barbara Kivimae Krimgold (eds). *Income, Socioeconomic Status, and Health: Exploring the Relationships.* Washington, D.C.: National Policy Association, and the Academy for Health Services Research and Policy, 2001.

Wilson, William Julius. *The Truly Disadvantaged.* Chicago: University of Chicago Press, 1987.

Wolf, Ann M., and Graham A. Colditz. "Current Estimates of the Economic Cost of Obesity in the United States." *Obesity Research* (1998): 6:97–106.

Wolf, Stewart and John G. Bruhn. *The Power of Clan. A 25-year Prospective Study of Roseto, Pennsylvania.* New Brunswick, NJ: Transaction Publishers, 1993.

Wolff, Edward N. *Top Heavy.* Expanded edition. New York: The New Press, 1996.

Young, Michael, and Peter Willmott. *Family and Friendship in East London.* London: Routledge and Kegan Paul, 1957.

Zunz, Oliver. *Why the American Century?* Chicago: Chicago University Press, 1999.

INDEX